Treatment of Asthma in Older Adults

Tolly E. G. Epstein • Sharmilee M. Nyenhuis
Editors

Treatment of Asthma in Older Adults

A Comprehensive, Evidence-Based Guide

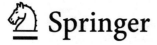 Springer

Editors
Tolly E. G. Epstein
Division of Immunology, Allergy
and Rheumatology
University of Cincinnati School of Medicine
Cincinnati, OH
USA

Sharmilee M. Nyenhuis
Division of Pulmonary, Critical Care, Sleep
and Allergy
University of Illinois at Chicago
Chicago, IL
USA

ISBN 978-3-030-20553-9   ISBN 978-3-030-20554-6   (eBook)
https://doi.org/10.1007/978-3-030-20554-6

This Springer imprint is published by the registered company Springer Nature Switzerland AG
The registered company address is: Gewerbestrasse 11, 6330 Cham, Switzerland

Preface

Asthma is a highly prevalent condition, affecting at least 26 million Americans, and the global prevalence of asthma continues to rise. Although asthma affects all age groups, adults age 65 years and older are disproportionately impacted by the disease. By 2030, the number of asthmatics age 65 years and older is expected to increase to five million in the USA alone [1]. Despite this high prevalence, the burden of asthma in older adults remains underappreciated. Compared to younger asthmatics, older asthmatics experience higher morbidity and mortality from asthma, a higher financial burden related to the disease, and poorer quality of life. This burden is compounded by a relative lack of research studies and clinical guidelines that specifically address issues related to asthma in older adults.

For the above reasons, Springer publishing approached us to ask that we compile a textbook that will assist clinicians who treat older adults with asthma. The result is the first comprehensive guidebook on the diagnosis and treatment of asthma in older adults in the past 20 years. This book is a summary of existing scientific evidence presented from the perspective of expert researchers and clinicians on asthma in older adults. The book is intended to be useful not only to physicians specializing in asthma but also to primary care physicians, students, case coordinators, and others who assist in the care of asthmatics age 65 years and older.

The book begins by defining the scope of the burden of asthma in older adults and explaining why asthma is more difficult to control in this age group. Included is a discussion regarding the challenges of diagnosis of asthma in older adults, such as the common misconception that asthma only begins in childhood, and difficulties with physician and patient self-perceptions of the disease. Methods to overcome challenges with objective testing in this age group are examined. Evidence-based recommendations regarding how to distinguish asthma from other common comorbidities are also provided.

The second part of the book is intended to provide methods to optimize effective treatment of asthma in older adults. This includes a discussion of how to overcome physical, cognitive, and emotional barriers to effective treatment in older asthmatics. A review of existing literature regarding the use of specific medications, including their efficacy and side effects, in older asthmatics is provided. This is coupled with a discussion of novel and alternative therapies for asthma, with specific reference to evidence for these treatments in older adults. Ways to overcome other challenges, including how to manage asthma in patients with multiple comorbidities and with different asthma phenotypes, are considered. Shared decision-making and strategies to optimize adherence in older adults are also discussed, along with specific recommendations for case coordinators and other nursing professionals caring for older asthmatics. Finally, an evidence-based review of the impact of indoor and outdoor environmental exposures, including allergens, pollutants, and infectious pathogens, on asthma in older adults is provided. This is followed by suggestions regarding how to control relevant environmental exposures.

It is our hope that this book will not only offer an evidence-based review of existing literature on asthma in older adults but also afford clinicians with tools that can immediately be used to help provide optimal care for this high-risk population.

Cincinnati, OH, USA   Tolly E. G. Epstein
Chicago, IL, USA   Sharmilee M. Nyenhuis

Reference

1. Stupka E, deShazo R. Asthma in seniors: part 1. Evidence for underdiagnosis, undertreatment, and increasing morbidity and mortality. Am J Med. 2009;122(1):6–11

Contents

Contributors

Alan P. Baptist, MD, MPH Division of Allergy and Clinical Immunology, Department of Internal Medicine, University of Michigan, Ann Arbor, MI, USA

Cheryl K. Bernstein, RN, BSN, CCRC Bernstein Clinical Research Center, LLC, Cincinnati, OH, USA

Don Bukstein, MD Allergy Asthma Sinus Center, Fitchburg and Milwaukee, Fitchburg, WI, USA

Ali Cheema, MD Pulmonary and Critical Care Medicine, Baylor College of Medicine, Houston, TX, USA

Rohit Divekar, MBBS, PhD Division of Allergic Diseases, Mayo Clinic, Rochester, MN, USA

Tolly E. G. Epstein, MD, MS FAAAAI Division of Immunology, Allergy, and Rheumatology, University of Cincinnati School of Medicine, Cincinnati, OH, USA

Pinkus Goldberg, MD, FAAAAI, FACAAI Indiana University School of Medicine, Indianapolis, IN, USA

Internal Medicine, Community Hospitals Health Care System of Indiana, Indianapolis, IN, USA

Allergy Partners of Central Indiana, Indianapolis, IN, USA

Nicola A. Hanania, MD, MS Pulmonary and Critical Care Medicine, Baylor College of Medicine, Houston, TX, USA

Dennis K. Ledford, MD Internal Medicine, James A. Haley VA Hospital, Tampa General Hospital, Moffitt Cancer Center, Advent Health, Tampa, FL, USA

Sameer K. Mathur, MD, PhD Department of Medicine, University of Wisconsin School of Medicine and Public Health, Madison, WI, USA

Anil Nanda, MD Asthma and Allergy Center, Lewisville and Flower Mound, TX, USA

Division of Allergy and Immunology, University of Texas Southwestern Medical Center, Dallas, TX, USA

Dharani K. Narendra, MD Pulmonary and Critical Care Medicine, Baylor College of Medicine, Houston, TX, USA

Sharmilee M. Nyenhuis, MD FAAAAI Division of Pulmonary, Critical Care, Sleep and Allergy, University of Illinois at Chicago, Chicago, IL, USA

Gayatri B. Patel, MD Division of Allergy and Immunology, Department of Medicine, Northwestern Feinberg School of Medicine, Chicago, IL, USA

Carol A. Saltoun, MD, MSCI Division of Allergy and Immunology, Department of Medicine, Northwestern Feinberg School of Medicine, Chicago, IL, USA

Joram S. Seggev, MD Internal Medicine, College of Medicine, Roseman University of Health Sciences, Las Vegas, NV, USA

Concettina (Tina) Tolomeo, DNP, APRN, FNP-BC, AE-C Yale Medicine and the Department of Pediatrics, Yale School of Medicine, New Haven, CT, USA

Anita N. Wasan, MD, FAAAAI Allergy and Asthma Center, McLean, VA, USA

Scope of the Burden of Asthma in Older Adults

1

Sharmilee M. Nyenhuis and Tolly E. G. Epstein

Asthma is commonly thought of as a disease of children and young adults, yet it affects a significant portion of the older adult ($\geq$65 years old) population [1]. The prevalence of current asthma in adults age 65 years and older in the USA is 7% based on the 2012 National Health Interview Survey (NHIS) [2]. Other countries, such as Portugal and Australia, have reported asthma prevalence as high as 11% in older adults [3]. By 2030, the number of asthmatics age 65 years and older is expected to increase to 5 million in the USA alone [4].

Despite increasing recognition of the high prevalence of asthma in older adults, the true burden of asthma in this growing population remains underappreciated. In the Cardiovascular Health Study, a large community-based cohort of older adults ($\geq$65 years old), participants were asked questions relevant to asthma with the goal to better understand the prevalence and effect of asthma in this population [5]. Based on participant responses, patients were categorized as having:

(a) Definite asthma: a positive response to the questions indicating that the patient had current asthma and that a physician confirmed the diagnosis
(b) Probable asthma: a history of wheezing in the past year associated with chest tightness or breathlessness

S. M. Nyenhuis (✉)
Division of Pulmonary, Critical Care, Sleep and Allergy, University of Illinois at Chicago, Chicago, IL, USA
e-mail: snyenhui@uic.edu

T. E. G. Epstein (✉)
Division of Immunology, Allergy, and Rheumatology, University of Cincinnati School of Medicine, Cincinnati, OH, USA
e-mail: epsteite@uc.edu

© Springer Nature Switzerland AG 2019
T. E. G. Epstein, S. M. Nyenhuis (eds.), *Treatment of Asthma in Older Adults*, https://doi.org/10.1007/978-3-030-20554-6_1

(c) Possible asthma: a positive response to the question, "Have you had wheezing or whistling in your chest at any time during the last 12 months?" and a positive response to three additional questions pertaining to nighttime asthma symptoms and triggers of asthma (exercise, dust, tobacco smoke, pollen, animals, seasons, bedding).

Smokers (current, recently quit <1 year ago, or ≥10 pack year smoking history) and those with a diagnosis of congestive heart failure were excluded. Four percent of subjects had definite asthma, 4% had probable asthma, and an additional 11% reported wheezing brought on by various exposures (possible asthma). Those with definite or probable asthma were more likely to be female than those without asthma. While the reasons for this are not well understood, this follows the shift seen in adolescence to a greater female prevalence of asthma and may be due to hormonal changes (menstrual cycle and menopause). The age of asthma onset in this cohort was spread evenly among decades. This has also been seen in other studies, where the incidence of new onset asthma remained the same throughout adult life [6]. Older adults with asthma in the Cardiovascular Health Study had more respiratory symptoms than younger asthmatics, with a two–fivefold increase in cough, phlegm, wheezing, and dyspnea.

Asthma mortality for all age groups steadily increased from 1980 until it peaked in 1998. Based on data from the Centers for Disease Control, there were 3518 deaths from asthma in the USA in 2016; most recent age-related data from 2014 indicated that 42.7% of those deaths were in adults age 65 years and older [7, 8] (Fig. 1.1). Another study found a threefold increase in the death rate among older adult asthmatics when compared to younger asthmatics [9–11]. Again, older women tend to have higher mortality rates than older men for unknown reasons.

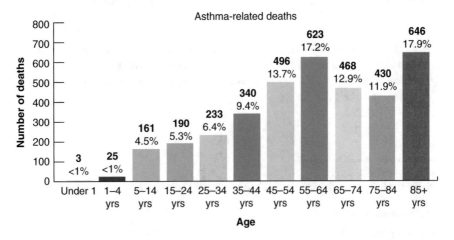

Fig. 1.1 Older adults are at the highest risk of fatality from asthma in the USA. Reproduced with permission from Asthma Capitals 2018: The Most Challenging Places to Live With Asthma. The Asthma and Allergy Foundation of America. Landover, MD. http://www.aafa.org/page/asthma-capitals.aspx

In addition to higher mortality rates, older adults may be impacted more by asthma in other ways. Older adults tend to be high utilizers of health-care resources. The National Ambulatory Medical Care Survey reported that patients 65 years or older have the second-highest rate of outpatient office visits after those aged 0–4 years and accounted for a greater proportion of hospitalizations (23%) than the size of its population (13%) would indicate [12]. Hospitalizations and emergency department visits are more common in older adults with asthma when compared to other adult cohorts. Older women are at greater risk than older men for hospitalization; the reasons for this are not well known [13]. Asthma significantly impacts quality of life in older adults. In the Cardiovascular Health Study, about one-third of patients with definite or probable asthma had significantly lower quality of life compared to those without asthma [5]. Kannan et al. examined predictors of poor asthma-related quality of life based on modified Asthma Quality of Life Questionnaire (mAQLQ) scores in 164 asthmatics aged 65 years and older [14]. They found that traffic-related air pollution exposure was the biggest risk factor for poor mAQLQ scores. Obesity, gastroesophageal reflux, non-atopic status, and an earlier onset of asthma were also significantly associated with poorer mAQLQ scores.

Underdiagnosis and underrecognition of asthma symptoms are significant reasons for poor asthma outcomes in the older adult population. The Respiratory Health in the Elderly Study found that only about half of older adults were correctly diagnosed with asthma in the past [15]. The 2007 Expert Panel Report on the Diagnosis and Management of Asthma recognizes that the diagnosis of asthma in older adults "poses a special challenge" [16]. There are both patient and health-care provider-related factors that contribute to the challenge of diagnosing asthma in older adults. Patients may deny having the disease or may account their breathing symptoms to aging. Older patients have a decreased perception of pulmonary symptoms, such as bronchoconstriction so may not be aware of their pulmonary symptoms [17]. Health-care providers may also underrecognize asthma symptoms as they may believe that adult-onset asthma is rare or the symptoms are due to aging. Underutilization of objective measures of lung function contributes to the underrecognition of asthma in older adults [5]. Older adults are able to perform good quality spirometry and DLCO, comparable to younger adults, and these objective tests should be utilized in the evaluation of respiratory symptoms [18]. Comorbid conditions are more common in older adults and may make it difficult for patients and providers to recognize the symptoms of asthma. For example, older adults with asthma may have a history of tobacco smoking which may make it difficult to distinguish which disease is producing the respiratory symptoms.

Even among older adults with an asthma diagnosis, inadequate treatment by health-care providers is commonly found. In the Cardiovascular Health Study, less than half of older adults with definite asthma had a rescue albuterol inhaler, and only 30% had an inhaled corticosteroid [5]. Sin and colleagues found that in older patients who were recently hospitalized for an acute asthma exacerbation, less than 50% were prescribed an ICS within 90 days of discharge [19]. Those at highest risk of not being on ICS were patients >80 years old, with high comorbidity index (>3), and were not receiving specialist follow-up care [19].

Multiple barriers to effective asthma treatment in older adults exist, but can be overcome through tailored strategies. One major barrier is a lack of good communication and shared goals between older patients and clinicians. To overcome this barrier, it is often useful to develop a team-based approach with the help of other health-care professionals. This will establish a forum to discuss misperceptions of disease, which are common in the older asthmatic population, and improve asthma-related health literacy [20]. Recognition by health-care providers of comorbid medical conditions that confound symptom identification and management, such as cognitive decline, depression, and cardiovascular disease, is also important [21]. Physical impairments and cognitive decline may influence the choice of therapies and teaching strategies for particular patients [22, 23]. Financial difficulties must also be taken into account when choosing therapies, as many older adults live on a fixed income and have difficulties affording medications. In addition, it is critical to understand that medication efficacy and side effects may vary greatly from younger populations [24]. Moreover, polypharmacy in this population frequently increases side effects and limits adherence [25, 26]. In addition to physiologic changes that occur with aging, older adults with asthma may also have different asthma phenotypes that may not respond as well to standard asthma medications [25]. Finally, older adult asthmatics may be more sensitive to the effects of environmental asthma triggers, including air pollutants and indoor allergens, which should be taken into account when developing treatment strategies [6, 14, 27].

The chapters that follow will discuss in great detail the above challenges in the diagnosis of asthma in older adults, and strategies to optimize the effective treatment of asthma in this population.

References

1. Busse PJ, Kilaru K. Complexities of diagnosis and treatment of allergic respiratory disease in the elderly. Drugs Aging. 2009;26(1):1–22.
2. Oraka E, et al. Asthma prevalence among US elderly by age groups: age still matters. J Asthma. 2012;49(6):593–9.
3. Pite H, et al. Prevalence of asthma and its association with rhinitis in the elderly. Respir Med. 2014;108(8):1117–26.
4. Stupka E, deShazo R. Asthma in seniors: part 1. Evidence for underdiagnosis, undertreatment, and increasing morbidity and mortality. Am J Med. 2009;122(1):6–11.
5. Enright P, et al. Underdiagnosis and undertreatment of asthma in the elderly. Chest. 1999;116(3):603–13.
6. Epstein TG, et al. Poor asthma control and exposure to traffic pollutants and obesity in older adults. Ann Allergy Asthma Immunol. 2012;108(6):423–428 e2.
7. Most recent asthma data from centers for disease control and prevention: US Department of Health & Human Services. Last Updated May 2018, Available from: https://www.cdc.gov/asthma/most_recent_data.htm. Accessed 26 Aug 2018.
8. Asthma capitals 2018: the most challenging places to live with asthma. 2018. Available from: http://www.aafa.org/page/asthma-capitals.aspx. Accessed 26 Aug 2018.

9. Moorman, J, et al. National Surveillance for Asthma — United States, 1980–2004, CDC, MMWR Surveillance Studies. October 19, 2007 / 56(SS08);1–14;18–54. https://www.cdc.gov/mmwr/preview/mmwrhtml/ss5608a1.htm. Accessed 17 May 2019.
10. Robin ED. Death from bronchial-asthma. Chest. 1988;93(3):614–8.
11. Slavin RG, et al. Asthma in older adults: observations from the epidemiology and natural history of asthma: outcomes and treatment regimens (TENOR) study. Ann Allergy Asthma Immunol. 2006;96(3):406–14.
12. Hanania NA, et al. Asthma in the elderly: current understanding and future research needs, a report of a National Institute on Aging (NIA) workshop. J Allergy Clin Immunol. 2011;128(3):S4–S24.
13. Barr RG, et al. Patient factors and medication guideline adherence among older women with asthma. Arch Intern Med. 2002;162(15):1761–8.
14. Kannan JA, et al. Significant predictors of poor quality of life in older asthmatics. Ann Allergy Asthma Immunol. 2015;115(3):198–204.
15. Bellia V, et al. Aging and disability affect misdiagnosis of COPD in elderly asthmatics – The SARA study. Chest. 2003;123(4):1066–72.
16. National Asthma Education and Prevention Program, full report of the expert panel: guidelines for the diagnosis and management of asthma (EPR-3; Source Document). National Heart, Lung and Blood Institute, 2007. http://www.nhlbi.nih.gov/guidelines/asthma/asthgdln.htm.
17. Ekici M, et al. Perception of bronchoconstriction in elderly asthmatics. J Asthma. 2001;38(8):691.
18. Haynes JM. Pulmonary function test quality in the elderly: a comparison with younger adults. Respir Care. 2014;59(1):16–21.
19. Sin DD, Tu JV. Underuse of inhaled steroid therapy in elderly patients with asthma. Chest. 2001;119(3):720–5.
20. O'Conor R, et al. A qualitative investigation of the impact of asthma and self-management strategies among older adults. J Asthma. 2017;54(1):39–45.
21. Bohmer MM, et al. Factors associated with generic health-related quality of life in adult asthma patients in Germany: cross-sectional study. J Asthma. 2017;54(3):325–34.
22. Melani AS, Paleari D. Maintaining control of chronic obstructive airway disease: adherence to inhaled therapy and risks and benefits of switching devices. COPD. 2016;13(2):241–50.
23. Melani AS, et al. Time required to rectify inhaler errors among experienced subjects with faulty technique. Respir Care. 2017;62(4):409–14.
24. de Roos EW, et al. Targeted therapy for older patients with uncontrolled severe asthma: current and future prospects. Drugs Aging. 2016;33(9):619–28.
25. Herscher ML, et al. Characteristics and outcomes of older adults with long-standing versus late-onset asthma. J Asthma. 2017;54(3):223–9.
26. Costello RW, et al. The seven stages of man: the role of developmental stage on medication adherence in respiratory diseases. J Allergy Clin Immunol Pract. 2016;4(5):813–20.
27. Epstein TG, et al. Chronic traffic pollution exposure is associated with eosinophilic, but not neutrophilic inflammation in older adult asthmatics. J Asthma. 2013;50(9):983–9.

Difficulties in Physician and Self-Perception of Asthma in Older Adults

Gayatri B. Patel and Carol A. Saltoun

According to the CDC asthma surveillance data from 2015, the national prevalence of asthma in those aged 65 years old and older was 6.6%. This is likely a gross underestimate given that asthma in older adults is frequently misdiagnosed, under-diagnosed, and undertreated [1, 2]. Reasons for this unrecognized disease burden in older adults have not been entirely elucidated; however, prior studies suggest that a driving factor is a failure of both physician and patient recognition of symptoms. Furthermore, there is no universal definition or established criteria for diagnosis of asthma in older adults. The focus of this chapter is to understand the barriers that prevent or delay the evaluation and subsequent diagnosis of asthma in older adults (see Table 2.1).

Patient-Specific Factors

Poor Perception

Older adults tend to have a decreased perception of their own airflow resistance which precludes them from recognizing respiratory abnormalities and discussing these problems with their physician [2, 3]. In separate studies performed by Connolly and Ekici, both authors showed that older adults with asthma have less

G. B. Patel · C. A. Saltoun (✉)
Division of Allergy and Immunology, Department of Medicine, Northwestern Feinberg School of Medicine, Chicago, IL, USA
e-mail: gayatri.patel@northwestern.edu; c-saltoun@northwestern.edu

© Springer Nature Switzerland AG 2019
T. E. G. Epstein, S. M. Nyenhuis (eds.), *Treatment of Asthma in Older Adults*,
https://doi.org/10.1007/978-3-030-20554-6_2

Table 2.1 Asthma in older adults: barriers and misperceptions

Patient-specific factors	Physician-specific factors
Misconception that dyspnea is due to aging	Misconception that dyspnea is due to aging
Attributes own symptoms to other existing comorbidities (i.e., COPD, heart failure)	Multiple patient comorbidities (i.e., COPD, heart failure) confound the work up for diagnosis
Decreased perception of symptoms with aging	Misconception that asthma is a pediatric disease and COPD is an adult disease
Poor memory recall of symptoms or describes non-specific symptoms	Lack of specialty referrals to pulmonology and/or allergy and immunology
Inability to perform correct technique for spirometry or PFTs (i.e., due to poor coordination, hearing difficulties, etc.)	Performing reliable spirometry and PFTs due to patient technique and effort. Difficulty with proper interpretation of testing
Concern with taking inhalers properly	Concern for polypharmacy and adherence
Depression, social isolation, difficulty attending appointments, fear of dying, or denial of symptoms	Lack of established criteria for diagnosis of asthma in older adults

awareness of bronchoconstriction despite having objective reduction in Forced Expiratory Volume in 1 second (FEV_1) compared to younger age groups with asthma [4, 5]. In another small, randomized double-blind crossover study of 20 young (mean age 27 years) and 20 older patients (mean age 83 years) without obvious confounding factors, subjects received isotonic saline as placebo vs nebulized distilled water. Results showed a significantly reduced number of coughs in older patients (5.58 coughs) compared to younger patients (15.4 coughs) suggesting a weaker cough reflex in older adults [6]. These changes could be from age-induced alterations to the sensory input from the lungs, particularly in the stretch receptors, or due to an age-related decrease in ventilation response with resulting hypoxia and hypercapnia. Poor perception or recognition by patients may manifest as reduced activity before complaints of subjective dyspnea occur [7, 8].

The lack of distinct symptoms can make it difficult for older patients to approach their physicians and adequately characterize their symptoms. This likely means that they will not vocalize their concerns unless explicitly asked by their provider. Older patients may also underestimate their respiratory symptoms if they are mostly sedentary and home bound. When performing an infrequent activity which causes dyspnea, cough, or chest tightness, the patient may relate it to being deconditioned. If a physician is suspicious that a patient has decreased self-perception of their respiratory symptoms, one approach can be to recommend patients to self-monitor with a peak flow meter. Peak flow monitoring is an Evidence Level A recommendation by the NIH National Asthma Education and Prevention Program asthma guidelines which advocate this approach in certain subgroup populations [9].

Psychosocial Factors

As discussed by other authors in this book, the role of depression in older adults with asthma deserves closer attention. It was shown in a National Health and

Nutrition Examination Survey (NHANES) study performed by Patel et al. that older asthmatics with depression had more emergency department and urgent care visits and limitation in activity, compared to older asthmatic adults without depression with similar spirometry values [10]. This suggests that undiagnosed or uncontrolled depression can make asthma diagnosis by physicians more difficult as depression may influence a patient's own perception of their own health and severity of symptoms [8]. Additionally, there is a positive correlation between asthma and depression contributing to poor quality of life which affects self-management [11]. Some older adults may fear end of life or illnesses that may place more restriction on them, making them reluctant to notify their provider [12]. Other contributing factors include: poor memory recall of symptoms, depression, social isolation, denial, and poor medical literacy which may prohibit older adults from seeking or eliciting medical advice [2, 12].

Patients with poor medical literacy will have difficulty in conveying their symptoms and concerns with their providers. In a large survey of asthma knowledge in 4066 adults ages 55–96 years with and without history of asthma, there was poor understanding of symptoms related to asthma. A large proportion were not able to identify that a cough at night (59.3% incorrect), chest tightness (47.9% incorrect), and shortness of breath (35.4% incorrect) were symptoms that could be related to asthma. Additionally, asthma knowledge worsened as age increased [13].

Older adults may not know what symptoms to discuss with their medical care provider in order to address their asthma needs. Providers who recognize this as a barrier can consider alternative management styles that can optimize care for older patients with asthma. For example, older patients with a physician diagnosis of asthma had improved control of their symptoms after a simple telephone intervention. Individuals in the intervention group were encouraged to discuss their symptomology with their primary care physicians. After two phone call interventions in 1 year, patients in the intervention group had a significant increase in the use of inhaled corticosteroids (ICS) [14]. This approach exemplifies how older patients require increased attention and engagement. Physicians may find that if they are having difficulty characterizing symptoms at one visit, it may be beneficial to perform telephone check-ins to further assess and clarify the diagnosis.

Physician-Specific Factors

Confounding Comorbidities

The symptoms of asthma in older adults are no different compared to younger populations of asthmatics and include shortness of breath, wheezing, chest tightness, and cough. The difficulty in easily attributing these symptoms to asthma in older adults is due to other age-related comorbidities that manifest similarly, whereas these symptoms tend to be more quickly linked to asthma in younger patients due to less confounding variables [15]. Depending on the symptom(s), physicians will consider what are more seemingly age-appropriate diagnoses including but not limited to coronary artery disease, congestive heart failure, chronic obstructive pulmonary disease (COPD), gastroesophageal reflux, anemia, tobacco use, obesity, or even aging itself. Moreover, multiple comorbidities with non-specific patterns of respiratory manifestations may make it nearly impossible to determine only one driving factor [15]. A common situation is that of a patient with a co-existing cardiac condition with respiratory symptoms who will have both conditions simultaneously or sequentially addressed. This can make it difficult to discern between disease entities [16]. For example, a patient may be started on a trial of low-dose Lasix and a daily controller inhaler making it difficult for physicians to distinguish which treatment had stronger impact.

When a pulmonary etiology is suspected as the cause of respiratory symptoms, it can be difficult to differentiate between COPD and asthma, as both have common, similar clinical features yet have distinct underlying immunological pathogenesis. A multicenter study performed in Italy evaluated the correct diagnosis (evaluated by history, physical examination, and spirometry) of asthma in 128 older adults (>65 years old) with asthma. It found that 68 (53.1%) patients had received the correct diagnosis of asthma, while 25 (19.5%) patients had an incorrect diagnosis of COPD, and 35 (27.3%) patients had not been given a prior diagnosis [17]. Identifiable reasons for *misdiagnosis* included older age followed by physical disability and an atypical pattern of asthma. The underlying rationale for these misconceptions is that asthma is a childhood disease associated with atopy which leads to early exclusion of the diagnosis, whereas COPD tends to be more fitting as a diagnosis for older adults. It should be noted that this was an older study when asthma-COPD overlap syndrome was not recognized. As more is learned about asthma-COPD overlap syndrome and increased awareness of late onset asthma, there will likely be more established criteria for recognizing asthma in advanced ages.

Attribution to Normal Aging

A likely notion by physicians and patients is that a decline in respiratory function can be attributed to aging alone so additional pathology such as asthma may not be considered [17]. There are, in fact, several factors that do contribute to physiological respiratory decline in older adults including (1) evidence that anatomical and physiological changes occur over time including progressive reduction in chest wall compliance, diaphragmatic muscle strength, and airway hyper-reactivity [18, 19]; (2) evidence of "senile lung" has been characterized in post-mortem analysis of lung tissue of individuals with no history of chronic lung disease which showed alveolar dilation without evidence of fibrosis [20]; and (3) the concept of immunosenescence or the age-related changes in innate and adaptive immune responses that lead to low-grade baseline systemic inflammation [18]. These known changes can make it difficult to differentiate "normal aging" versus a disease state; however, one can argue that certain symptoms such as dyspnea on exertion, acute shortness of breath, and wheezing should not be attributed as normal.

Unaware of Risk Factors

The physician's awareness and ability to identify risk factors for asthma in older adults can be tremendously helpful in leading to a diagnosis of asthma, although none of these risk factors have strong specificity. Preceding or concomitant viral illness related to development of respiratory symptoms should be investigated, as the relationship between viral triggers and asthma has been well documented in children [21]. Additionally, physicians should be suspicious if a patient gives the history of aspirin and/or non-steroidal anti-inflammatory drugs (NSAIDs) causing respiratory distress. This could suggest underlying asthma-exacerbated respiratory disease, a form of asthma, and should be worked up if appropriate. There is a link suggesting that older adults with major depressive disorder are at higher risk for subsequent adult onset asthma [22]. Another unique population that may be at relatively higher risk for asthma is post-menopausal women on hormone replacement therapy (HRT) [23]. One study showed post-menopausal women on HRT have 2.24-fold increased risk of having new-onset asthma [24]. The link between post-menopausal females on HRT and risk of asthma is based only on association; further studies are needed to verify a causal relationship. Lacking knowledge of what risk factors exist for asthma in older adults makes it less likely that a physician will initiate an appropriate work up when an older adult presents with non-specific respiratory symptoms. Physicians need to maintain a high degree of vigilance and discernment when managing an older adult with new respiratory symptoms. In addition, experts need to continue to educate primary care physicians and trainees on risk factors and limitations when evaluating these patients.

Diagnostic Challenges

Physicians face challenges with diagnostic testing when evaluating asthma in older adults, due to both underutilization of testing and difficulty with interpreting tests. In a population-based study of 98 individuals with new-onset asthma over the age of 65, only 43% had at least one spirometry test and only 24% had at least one office peak flow [25]. A relatively recent study in Ontario, Canada, looked at a larger cohort of 465,866 patients with asthma of all ages. The study showed that objective pulmonary function testing (PFT) is still underutilized in the diagnosis of asthma; PFTs were done 42%, 29%, and 9.5% of the time in patients aged 70–79, 80–89, and 90–99 years old, respectively [26]. Both studies reflect the ongoing underutilization in diagnostic testing for asthma in older adults and also suggest that serial monitoring is underperformed. A reasonable explanation for this may be that physicians may not consider results reliable given that effort-dependent maneuvers may be reduced in older adults due to frailty, motor comorbidities such as Parkinson's disease, or cognitive impairment. Patients may not be able to efficiently perform forced expiratory maneuver, or sensory deficits such as deafness, cataracts, or dentures may limit the patient's performance [27].

When successful testing is performed, interpreting results can be the next hurdle. Prior studies have shown that there is normal reduction in FEV_1 due to aging, thus using standardized FEV_1/forced vital capacity (FVC) <70% may not be appropriate for diagnosing older individuals and could even lead to overdiagnosis [28]. Some experts advocate using FEV_1/FEV_6 with cutoff of 73% predicted or using the lowest 5% as a substitute for FEV_1/FVC 70% predicted which may provide more utility in diagnosing obstruction in older adults [29]. When obstruction is obvious such as the presence of air trapping or lack of reversibility with bronchodilator, it is important that the physician includes COPD or *severe* asthma in the differential [15, 30]. Severe asthma can present as fixed obstruction in cases where diagnosis has been delayed. This may mean that reversibility was not captured earlier on in the disease course and has already progressed to irreversible obstruction. Another reason for lack of reversibility may be due to age-related impairment in beta adrenoceptor responsiveness and not necessarily due to severe progression of asthma [31]. This distinction requires the physician to obtain a thorough history with aid of other laboratory parameters such as diffusing capacity for carbon monoxide and exhaled nitric oxide to prevent the incorrect label of COPD [32]. Overall, when testing is performed, it is crucial to remain open to the differential diagnosis and not make hasty diagnoses based on prior pattern recognition.

There are no other standardized, accepted tools used for diagnosing asthma in older adults. Although the use of exhaled nitric oxide has been extensively studied as a potential marker for assessing asthma in older adults, it is not currently established as standard for diagnostics. Methacholine challenge could be utilized more in older adults to assist with diagnosis, but this may be less accurate, and there would be increased concern for severe airway narrowing as healthy older individuals show increased airway hyper-responsiveness [19]. Skin testing is utilized more in younger patients suspected of having asthma but is not strongly supported to be useful in older adults. There is conflicting evidence on the link between asthma and IgE-positive aeroallergen testing in older adults with asthma [33]. This is discussed further in a subsequent chapter.

Physicians may empirically prescribe inhaled corticosteroids as a diagnostic strategy by testing for therapeutic effect based on symptoms and FEV_1 improvement. Before proceeding with this type of diagnostic therapeutic trial, it is important to understand what phenotypes of asthma respond well to ICS. In a study by Meyers et al., healthy non-asthmatic individuals aged 64–83 were found to have increased neutrophils, IL-8, and neutrophil granular constituents in bronchoalveolar lavage fluid compared to younger cohorts who had more eosinophilic, Th2 immune cells. This suggests that older adults with asthma may have a more neutrophilic-predominant phenotype or non-eosinophilic subtype. The neutrophilic subtype has been shown to have less of a response to ICS [34]. This suggests that an unsuccessful empiric trial of ICS treatment may falsely rule out asthma when it is possible that the problem is in fact driven by refractory neutrophilic asthma.

Lack of Specialty Referrals

Lastly, another barrier may be that older adults with respiratory symptoms of unclear etiology are not being appropriately referred to specialists who have expertise in managing this specific patient population. One study looked at referral patterns to subspecialists for patients with a history concerning for asthma. This study identified 98 older adult patients with onset of asthma after age 65 years, and found that only 15% had been referred to allergy, and 20% had been referred to pulmonology. This suggests that if any work up or diagnostics were performed, they were more commonly carried out by the primary care provider [25]. Primary care providers may not be equipped with the specialized knowledge and/or tools such as spirometry to identify asthma in older adults. With the recent availability of several biologics for the treatment of severe asthma, it is becoming more and more important to assess these patients' asthma phenotype for appropriate, tailored care. Encouraging referrals to specialists should be emphasized in order to address this gap in care of asthma in older adults.

In conclusion, a growing body of evidence shows that there are both patient- and physician-specific factors that lead to unrecognized or delayed presentations of asthma in older adults. It will require a concerted effort among physicians to address the large unmet need of appropriately identifying and managing these patients. Specific recommendations are provided in Table 2.2. Support groups and telephone interventions may provide patients with a channel to understand and characterize their respiratory symptoms. Physicians should understand limitations to diagnostics and remain cognizant of patients' psychosocial factors when considering asthma as a diagnosis. A multifaceted approach that promotes active engagement from patient, family, and other medical care providers is paramount.

Table 2.2 Recommendations for improving recognition of asthma in older patients

Increase education to primary care physicians on awareness of late onset asthma in older adults and associated risk factors

Encourage increased utilization of specialist referrals

Understand the limitations of current diagnostic approaches when used in older adults

Consider home peak flow monitoring to further evaluate respiratory limitations

Address underlying cognitive dysfunction or depression with appropriate services

Encourage frequent, active engagement from patient and family. Consider telephone calls or more frequent office visits for complex patients and/or those with multiple comorbidities

Encourage tools that promote self-management of illness such as support groups

References

1. Most recent asthma data, 2018. [Internet]. Atlanta. Centers for Disease Control and Prevention 2018 [cited 2018 March 23]. Available from https://www.cdcgov/asthma/most_recent_data. htm
2. Gillman A, Douglass JA. Asthma in the elderly. Asia Pac Allergy. 2012;2(2):101–8.
3. Allen S, Khattan A. The airflow resistance sensing threshold during tidal breathing rises in old age in patients with asthma. Age Ageing. 2012;41:557–60.
4. Connolly MJ, Crowley JJ, Charan NB, Nielson CP, Vestal RE. Reduced subjective awareness of bronchoconstriction provoked by methacholine in elderly asthmatic and normal subjects as measured on a simple awareness scale. Thorax. 1992;47(6):410–3.
5. Ekici M, Apan A, Ekici A, Erdemoglu AK. Perception of bronchoconstriction in elderly asthmatics. J Asthma. 2001;38(8):691–6.
6. Newnham D, Hamilton SJ. Sensitivity of the cough reflex in young and elderly subjects. Age Ageing. 1997;26(3):185–8.
7. Mahler DA. Evaluation of dyspnea in the elderly. Clin Geriatr Med. 2017;33(4):503–21.
8. Madeo J, Li Z, Frieri M. Asthma in the geriatric population. Allergy Asthma Proc. 2013;34(5):427–33.
9. National Asthma Education and Prevention Program Expert Panel Report 3. 2007 [Internet]. Bethesda: National Heart, Lung and Blood Institute 2007. p. 1–60. [cited 2018 March 23]. Available from: https://www.nhlbinihgov/files/docs/guidelines/asthsumm.pdf
10. Patel PO, Patel MR, Baptist AP. Depression and asthma outcomes in older adults: results from the National Health and Nutrition Examination Survey. J Allergy Clin Immunol Pract. 2017;5(6):1691–7 e1.
11. Ross JA, Yang Y, Song PX, Clark NM, Baptist AP. Quality of life, health care utilization, and control in older adults with asthma. J Allergy Clin Immunol Pract. 2013;1(2):157–62.
12. Braman SS. Asthma in the elderly. Clin Geriatr Med. 2017;33(4):523–37.
13. Evers U, Jones SC, Caputi P, Iverson D. The asthma knowledge and perceptions of older Australian adults: implications for social marketing campaigns. Patient Educ Couns. 2013;91(3):392–9.
14. Patel RR, Saltoun CA, Grammer LC. Improving asthma care for the elderly: a randomized controlled trial using a simple telephone intervention. J Asthma. 2009;46(1):30–5.
15. Hanania NA, King MJ, Braman SS, Saltoun C, Wise RA, Enright P, et al. Asthma in the elderly: current understanding and future research needs – a report of a National Institute on Aging (NIA) workshop. J Allergy Clin Immunol. 2011;128(3 Suppl):S4–24.
16. Baptist AP, Deol BB, Reddy RC, Nelson B, Clark NM. Age-specific factors influencing asthma management by older adults. Qual Health Res. 2010;20(1):117–24.
17. Bellia V, Battaglia S, Catalano F, Scichilone N, Incalzi RA, Imperiale C, et al. Aging and disability affect misdiagnosis of COPD in elderly asthmatics: the SARA study. Chest. 2003;123(4):1066–72.
18. Dunn RM, Busse PJ, Wechsler ME. Asthma in the elderly and late-onset adult asthma. Allergy. 2018;73(2):284–94.
19. Scichilone N, Messina M, Battaglia S, Catalano F, Bellia V. Airway hyperresponsiveness in the elderly: prevalence and clinical implications. Eur Respir J. 2005;25(2):364–75.
20. Verbeken EK, Cauberghs M, Mertens I, Clement J, Lauweryns JM, Van de Woestijne KP. The senile lung. Comparison with normal and emphysematous lungs. 2. Functional aspects. Chest. 1992;101(3):800–9.
21. Proud D, Chow CW. Role of viral infections in asthma and chronic obstructive pulmonary disease. Am J Respir Cell Mol Biol. 2006;35(5):513–8.
22. Shen TC, Lin CL, Liao CH, Wei CC, Sung FC, Kao CH. Major depressive disorder is associated with subsequent adult-onset asthma: a population-based cohort study. Epidemiol Psychiatr Sci. 2017;26(6):664–71.

23. Zemp E, Schikowski T, Dratva J, Schindler C, Probst-Hensch N. Asthma and the menopause: a systematic review and meta-analysis. Maturitas. 2012;73(3):212–7.
24. Barr RG, Wentowski CC, Grodstein F, Somers SC, Stampfer MJ, Schwartz J, et al. Prospective study of postmenopausal hormone use and newly diagnosed asthma and chronic obstructive pulmonary disease. Arch Intern Med. 2004;164(4):379–86.
25. Bauer BA, Reed CE, Yunginger JW, Wollan PC, Silverstein MD. Incidence and outcomes of asthma in the elderly. Chest. 111(2):303–10.
26. Gershon AS, Victor JC, Guan J, Aaron SD, To T. Pulmonary function testing in the diagnosis of asthma: a population study. Chest. 2012;141(5):1190–6.
27. Chotirmall SH, Watts M, Branagan P, Donegan CF, Moore A, McElvaney NG. Diagnosis and management of asthma in older adults. J Am Geriatr Soc. 2009;57(5):901–9.
28. Hansen JE, Sun X-G, Wasserman K. Spirometric criteria for airway obstruction. Chest. 131(2):349–55.
29. Melbye H, Medbo A, Crockett A. The FEV1/FEV6 ratio is a good substitute for the FEV1/FVC ratio in the elderly. Prim Care Respir J. 2006;15(5):294–8.
30. Scichilone N, Pedone C, Battaglia S, Sorino C, Bellia V. Diagnosis and management of asthma in the elderly. Eur J Intern Med. 2014;25(4):336–42.
31. Gupta P, O'Mahony MS. Potential adverse effects of bronchodilators in the treatment of airways obstruction in older people: recommendations for prescribing. Drugs Aging. 2008;25(5):415–43.
32. Fabbri LM, Romagnoli M, Corbetta L, Casoni G, Busljetic K, Turato G, et al. Differences in airway inflammation in patients with fixed airflow obstruction due to asthma or chronic obstructive pulmonary disease. Am J Respir Crit Care Med. 2003;167(3):418–24.
33. Scichilone N, Callari A, Augugliaro G, Marchese M, Togias A, Bellia V. The impact of age on prevalence of positive skin prick tests and specific IgE tests. Respir Med. 2011;105(5):651–8.
34. Wenzel SE. Asthma: defining of the persistent adult phenotypes. Lancet (London, England). 2006;368(9537):804–13.

Objective Testing for Asthma in Older Adults

3

Rohit Divekar

Defining Asthma and Its Implications to Objective Diagnostic Testing in Older Adults

Asthma is characterized by a functional impairment of airflow due to variable and reversible obstruction in lung airways accompanied by inflammation and other adaptive changes [1]. There are physical and mechanical changes that occur in the lung and the airways in asthma. These include (1) a reduction in airway caliber due to both luminal reduction in cross-sectional area of conducting airways and (2) intra-luminal changes such as the presence of intra-luminal debris (epithelial cells, other inflammatory cells, and/or intra-luminal mucous plugs). The biological alterations of asthma include an increase in inflammatory processes in the airway, increased mucus production, increased mucus-secreting cell hyperplasia, and adaptive changes to airway smooth muscle [1]. Given these numerous mechanical-physical and biological-chemical alterations in the lungs of patients with asthma, the objective measures of asthma should attempt to define the degree of change for those specific parameters.

In parallel, other biological and physical processes operate in the lungs of older adults due to: (1) age-related changes [2]; (2) the influence of other pulmonary comorbidities on lung function such as chronic obstructive pulmonary disease (COPD); and [3] overall health status. In addition to the age-related changes, Baptist et al. reported key differences among older adults with asthma based on the duration of asthma, comorbidities, and fixed airway obstruction [4]. This superimposition of "heterogeneity" on "age-related" changes in the setting of "asthma-related" changes in the lung may add complexity in the assessment of asthma in older adults. The underlying qualifier of "aged-lung" would in part affect the interpretation and clinical implications of "asthma-specific" objective testing. Objective tests used to diagnose asthma in older adults are for the most part similar to testing in younger adults,

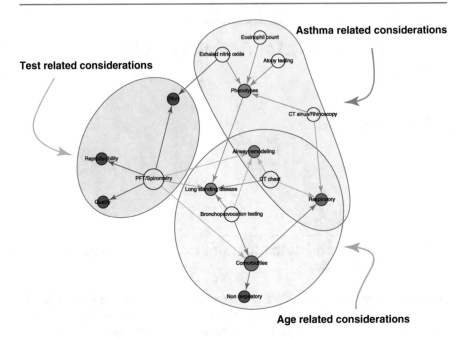

Fig. 3.1 A network linkage diagram illustrating the relationship between asthma-related factors, age-related factors, and specific test-related factors. Clear nodes represent objective measures used for assessment of asthma

but the effect of aging on test outcome should be considered [5] (Fig. 3.1). This chapter will characterize common and unique aspects of objective testing in asthma as they pertain to older adults.

Utilizing the Subjective Asthma Assessment and Objective Testing

Before objective testing in asthma is discussed, it is important to consider the subjective assessment of asthma control using validated tools such as the asthma control test or asthma control questionnaire (Fig. 3.2). Due to the long-standing nature of asthma in some older adults, the subjective assessment of asthma control may not accurately estimate the degree of asthma burden. Asthma-related quality of life questionnaires such as the mini Asthma quality of life questionnaire (mAQLQ) in older asthmatics have been shown to mirror those in younger populations, and are predictive of other measurements of asthma control, verifying that the such standardized tools may be appropriate for older adults with asthma [6]. If the older adult indicates that they "feel asthma is controlled" and the spirometric or function assessment is congruent with their subjective assessment, then no additional changes in therapy may be necessary. If the symptoms are controlled and stable for a long time, then de-escalation of therapy may even be considered. If the older adult indicates that their "asthma is not well controlled" and objective spirometric or functional

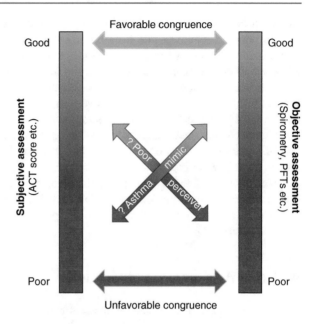

Fig. 3.2 Objective tests in asthma and their relationship to subjective asthma burden in older adults. The diagram illustrates four possible scenarios relating objective asthma tests with subjective asthma control

assessment is congruent with their subjective assessment, then optimization of medical therapy and/or assessment of compliance and technique may be necessary.

The objective tests are indispensable when the subjective assessment of asthma control is not congruent with objective data [7]. If the patient indicates that their "asthma is controlled" but the objective assessment is not in alignment with their subjective assessment, then exploring whether a perception bias exists may be important. Long-standing asthma patients, especially older adults, may perceive asthma symptoms as "controlled," yet their symptoms are far from controlled. Including the objective data in discussion of ongoing care may motivate them to be cognizant of the "real" burden of disease. Older adults often poorly perceive acute changes in airway caliber. For example, Connolly et al. showed that older adults with asthma were less aware of the reduction in forced expiratory volume in 1 second (FEV_1) as provoked by a bronchial provocation with methacholine [8]. Alternatively, if the patient indicates that his/her asthma is "not controlled" and the spirometric or function assessment is normal or within reference values, then other conditions that mimic poor asthma control (cardiac disease, vocal cord dysfunction, maladaptive breathing patterns, anxiety, etc.) may need to be evaluated [9].

Tests of Pulmonary Function and Airflow Limitation

Pulmonary Function Tests and Spirometry in Older Adults

When considering spirometry in older adults, the quality of the effort and age-adjusted values are essential, especially during interpretation of the test results [10]. The SARA (acronym from "SAlute Respiratoria nell'Anziano" = "Respiratory

Health in the Elderly") study identified a few specific patient-related factors that lead to poor acceptability rate for spirometry performance in older adults [11]. These included cognitive impairment, shorter 6-minute walk distance, and lower educational level. Cognitive impairment may relate to difficulty with performing complex tasks. A shorter 6-minute walk distance may reflect poor lung function with inability to sustain quality maneuvers. In the same study, male gender and advanced age were risk factors for poorer reproducibility of FEV_1 [11]. Cumulatively, these factors contributed to older adults having difficulty in performing the complex task of a pulmonary function test. These factors led to issues with comprehending directions, following instructions, coordination, and physical inability to meet the physical demand of the spirometric effort. However, despite the technical challenges of performing this task in older adults, reliable data can be obtained if special attention to the technique and execution of spirometry testing in older adults is made a priority [11].

Peak Flow Assessment in Older Adults

Assessment of peak flow in older adults is affected by effort-dependent parameters and would be expected to follow similar limitations as spirometry. In fact, although others have disagreed, Buist et al. report that there was no advantage to peak flow monitoring over symptom monitoring as an asthma management strategy for older adults [12]. The patients in this study had moderate to severe asthma and peak expiratory flow (PEF) testing used in a comprehensive asthma management program [12]. In a large community sample of older subjects, Enright et al. reported that mean PEF at home was an accurate reflection of PEF determined by clinic spirometric methods. The lability of PEF was also thought to demonstrate a greater association with asthma [13]. The lability of the PEF likely reflects the variable airflow limitation seen in asthma. However, the 2007 expert panel report-3 does recommend spirometry for diagnostic purposes rather than measurements by a peak flow meter in the clinician's office due to the wide variability in published predicted peak expiratory flow (PEF) reference values [14]. The report suggests using specific symptoms and peak expiratory flow (PEF) measurement for monitoring of asthma, and this would also be applicable to older adults [14].

Assessment of Bronchial Hyperresponsiveness

Bronchial provocation testing is an important component of asthma diagnosis. This test assesses airway reactivity in the form of hyperresponsiveness to provocation with inhaled agents either by direct provocation with histamine or methacholine or an indirect provocation with mannitol [15]. Regardless of the agent employed to perform the testing, certain contraindications to the test make them especially relevant to the older adult population [16]. Older adults have a greater prevalence of cardiac and vascular comorbidities such as myocardial infarction (MI) or stroke. A history of recent MI or stroke is an absolute contraindication to bronchial provocation testing [16]. Uncontrolled hypertension and known aortic aneurysm are also contraindications. Presence of ocular and ophthalmic comorbidities in older adults (glaucoma, cataracts, etc.) may put them at higher risk of recently having eye surgery, which is a contraindication for this test. Additional relative contraindications may also exist such as being unable to perform the maneuvers necessary for a satisfactory test due to physical limitation or cognitive decline [16].

Assessment of Airway Inflammation

Exhaled nitric oxide (eNO) has been shown to be a non-invasive surrogate of eosinophilic airway inflammation [17]. Respiratory maneuvers affect the outcome of eNO testing, and respiratory maneuvers may complicate interpretation of tests in older adults [18]. It is therefore recommended to consider eNO testing before spirometry in patients with asthma of any age. In a random adult population study, age was also independently and positively associated with eNO levels; subjects >64 years of age had 40% higher eNO values as compared to their younger adult counterparts [19]. However, among young and older adults specifically with asthma, there were no age-related differences in eNO levels in one study [20]. Nonetheless, there were differences in normative values for eNO based on age in a cross-sectional analysis of unselected who were lifelong non-smokers, and free of asthma, and other respiratory conditions and symptoms up to 79 years old from the National Health and Nutrition Examination Survey (2007–2010). In this study, geometric mean FeNO levels increased with age, from 8.3, 12.1, and 16.2 parts per billion (ppb) for males in the 6–11, 12–19, and 20–79 year age ranges, respectively. There were similar increases from 8.4, 10.9, and 12.6 ppb in the respective age groups in females. The highest FeNO levels were noted among 60–79-year-olds at 17.3 ppb, overall [21].

Other Objective Tests that Relate to Asthma Diagnosis

Blood Eosinophil Count

Age-related changes in eosinophil functional effects, such as reduction in eosinophil degranulation in response to IL-5 stimulation, have been reported [22]. While some functional aspects may be different in older adults, a subphenotype characterization based on eosinophil counts may still be applicable in this age group. Biological medications such as mepolizumab and other anti-IL-5 antibodies have been shown to best demonstrate effect in subjects with eosinophil-dependent disease. Both MENSA (Mepolizumab as Adjunctive Therapy in Patients with Severe Asthma) and SIRIUS (Steroid Reduction with Mepolizumab Study) clinical trials showed benefit of IL-5 antagonist mepolizumab, which included older patients in the study (upper range 82 years and 74 years, respectively) [23, 24].

Allergy Tests for Atopy/Sensitization

Allergy tests in older adults may suggest the presence of atopic sensitization as a contributor to asthma pathogenesis. However, interpretation of skin tests and IgE tests in older adults has their own challenges, accounting for both false negatives and false positives. Age-related skin changes may make interpretation of skin test results challenging due to super imposition of photo-damage, although both processes are distinct [25]. A number of studies have demonstrated that atopy, as tested by skin prick tests and specific serum IgE, declines with age [20, 26]. This may be a result of immunosenescence, genetic and epigenetic changes in skin constituents, local changes in vasculature, changes in the skin such as amount of dermal collagen, composition of inflammatory and other cell types in the dermal layer, and other comorbid skin conditions [27, 28]. False positives may be a consequence of other inflammatory dermatoses, and a careful assessment of the skin prior to testing is essential. If clinical suspicion is high and there is a temporal relationship between asthma exacerbations and the presence of allergic triggers, then in vitro assays may be performed in cases in which skin testing cannot be performed. Allergen positivity in older adults does exist; if present in the context of asthma, it should be addressed by offering environmental modifications for reduction of allergen exposure, appropriate medications, and possibly immunotherapy [29].

Objective Tests for Chronic Inflammatory Sinus Disease

Radiological tests such as CT scan of paranasal sinuses and direct visualization with rhinolaryngoscopy are essential for diagnosis of chronic inflammatory sinus disease. In a survey-based postal questionnaire conducted by the Global Allergy and Asthma Network of Excellence (GALEN) study, the association with asthma was stronger in those reporting both chronic rhinosinusitis and allergic rhinitis [30]. In a self-reported questionnaire, the estimated prevalence of current chronic rhinosinusitis showed an age-dependent increase in weighted prevalence from 18 to 59 years of age (15.9%) after which there was a decline to 6.8% after 69 years of age [31]. Uncontrolled chronic rhinosinusitis can affect symptom assessment of asthma. Management of chronic rhinosinusitis has also been demonstrated to impact asthma quality of life [32]. Due to the age-associated changes in prevalence of chronic rhinosinusitis [31, 33] and the strong association of chronic rhinosinusitis with asthma [34], it is reasonable to consider rhinolaryngoscopy or CT sinus examination as objective testing in the older adult with asthma, especially if they have sinonasal complaints that are not consistent with allergic rhinitis alone.

CT and X-Ray Imaging of Chest

Radiological testing such as X-ray and CT scans of the chest are important for diagnosis of other pulmonary disorders, as well as non-pulmonary conditions affecting the lung. Moreover, CT scan of the chest can delineate pulmonary architecture with a high degree of resolution. Lung volumes and anatomic changes such as those suggestive of air trapping can be used to infer lung function in older adults [5]. CT imaging of older adults with asthma has revealed greater airway wall thickness compared to younger adults with asthma, and may be a useful adjunct to other objective testing in older adults [20]. Given that CT imaging is not a standard diagnostic tool for asthma, it may be best left to specialist interpretation at this time.

References

1. Kumar RK, Jeffery PK. Pathology of asthma. In: Chapter 60: Middleton's Allergy: Principles and Practice. 8th ed. Philadephia: Saunders, an imprint of Elsevier; 2014. p. 986–999.
2. Sharma G, Goodwin J. Effect of aging on respiratory system physiology and immunology. Clin Interv Aging. 2006;1(3):253.
3. Postma DS, Rabe KF. The asthma-COPD overlap syndrome. N Engl J Med. 2015;373(13):1241–9.
4. Baptist AP, Hao W, Karamched KR, Kaur B, Carpenter L, Song PX. Distinct asthma phenotypes among older adults with asthma. J Allergy Clin Immunol Pract. 2018;6(1):244–9. e2.
5. Skloot GS, Busse PJ, Braman SS, Kovacs EJ, Dixon AE, Vaz Fragoso CA, et al. An official American Thoracic Society workshop report: evaluation and management of asthma in the elderly. Ann Am Thorac Soc. 2016;13(11):2064–77.
6. Kannan JA, Bernstein DI, Bernstein CK, Ryan PH, Bernstein JA, Villareal MS, et al. Significant predictors of poor quality of life in older asthmatics. Ann Allergy Asthma Immunol. 2015;115(3):198–204.
7. Harrison B. Difficult asthma in adults: recognition and approaches to management. Intern Med J. 2005;35(9):543–7.
8. Connolly M, Crowley J, Charan N, Nielson C, Vestal R. Reduced subjective awareness of bronchoconstriction provoked by methacholine in elderly asthmatic and normal subjects as measured on a simple awareness scale. Thorax. 1992;47(6):410–3.
9. King CS, Moores LK. Clinical asthma syndromes and important asthma mimics. Respir Care. 2008;53(5):568–82.
10. Quanjer PH, Stanojevic S, Cole TJ, Baur X, Hall GL, Culver BH, et al. Multi-ethnic reference values for spirometry for the 3–95-yr age range: the global lung function 2012 equations. Eur Respir J. 2012;40(6):1324–43.
11. Bellia V, Pistelli R, Catalano F, Antonelli-Incalzi R, Grassi V, Melillo G, et al. Quality control of spirometry in the elderly. The SA.R.A. study. SAlute Respiration nell'Anziano = Respiratory Health in the Elderly. Am J Respir Crit Care Med. 2000;161(4 Pt 1): 1094–100.
12. Buist AS, Vollmer WM, Wilson SR, Frazier EA, Hayward AD. A randomized clinical trial of peak flow versus symptom monitoring in older adults with asthma. Am J Respir Crit Care Med. 2006;174(10):1077–87.
13. Enright PL, McClelland RL, Buist AS, Lebowitz MD, Group CHSR. Correlates of peak expiratory flow lability in elderly persons. Chest. 2001;120(6):1861–8.
14. National Institutes of Health, National Heart Lung and Blood Institute, National Asthma Education and Prevention Program. Expert panel report 3: guidelines for the diagnosis and management of asthma, August 2007. Available at https://www.nhlbi.nih.gov/files/docs/guidelines/asthsumm.pdf. Accessed 18 Dec 2018.
15. Brannan JD, Anderson SD, Perry CP, Freed-Martens R, Lassig AR, Charlton B. The safety and efficacy of inhaled dry powder mannitol as a bronchial provocation test for airway hyperresponsiveness: a phase 3 comparison study with hypertonic (4.5%) saline. Respir Res. 2005;6(1):144.

16. Crapo R. Guidelines for methacholine and exercise challenge testing-1999. This official statement of the American Thoracic Society was adopted by the ATS Board of Directors, July 1999. Am J Respir Crit Care Med. 2000;161:309–29.
17. Dweik RA, Boggs PB, Erzurum SC, Irvin CG, Leigh MW, Lundberg JO, et al. An official ATS clinical practice guideline: interpretation of exhaled nitric oxide levels (FENO) for clinical applications. Am J Respir Crit Care Med. 2011;184(5):602–15.
18. American Thoracic Society, European Respiratory Society. ATS/ERS recommendations for standardized procedures for the online and offline measurement of exhaled lower respiratory nitric oxide and nasal nitric oxide, 2005. Am J Respir Crit Care Med. 2005;171(8):912–30.
19. Olin A-C, Rosengren A, Thelle DS, Lissner L, Bake B, Torén K. Height, age, and atopy are associated with fraction of exhaled nitric oxide in a large adult general population sample. Chest. 2006;130(5):1319–25.
20. Inoue H, Niimi A, Takeda T, Matsumoto H, Ito I, Matsuoka H, et al. Pathophysiological characteristics of asthma in the elderly: a comprehensive study. Ann Allergy Asthma Immunol. 2014;113(5):527–33.
21. Brody DJ, Zhang X, Kit BK, Dillon CF. Reference values and factors associated with exhaled nitric oxide: US youth and adults. Respir Med. 2013;107(11):1682–91.
22. Mathur SK, Schwantes EA, Jarjour NN, Busse WW. Age-related changes in eosinophil function in human subjects. Chest. 2008;133(2):412–9.
23. Ortega HG, Liu MC, Pavord ID, Brusselle GG, FitzGerald JM, Chetta A, et al. Mepolizumab treatment in patients with severe eosinophilic asthma. N Engl J Med. 2014;371(13):1198–207.
24. Bel EH, Wenzel SE, Thompson PJ, Prazma CM, Keene ON, Yancey SW, et al. Oral glucocorticoid-sparing effect of mepolizumab in eosinophilic asthma. N Engl J Med. 2014;371(13):1189–97.
25. King MJ, Lockey RF. Allergen prick-puncture skin testing in the elderly. Drugs Aging. 2003;20(14):1011–7.
26. Scichilone N, Callari A, Augugliaro G, Marchese M, Togias A, Bellia V. The impact of age on prevalence of positive skin prick tests and specific IgE tests. Respir Med. 2011;105(5):651–8.
27. Gronniger E, Weber B, Heil O, Peters N, Stab F, Wenck H, et al. Aging and chronic sun exposure cause distinct epigenetic changes in human skin. PLoS Genet. 2010;6(5):e1000971.
28. Quan T, Fisher GJ. Role of age-associated alterations of the dermal extracellular matrix microenvironment in human skin aging: a mini-review. Gerontology. 2015;61(5):427–34.
29. Brozek JL, Bousquet J, Baena-Cagnani CE, Bonini S, Canonica GW, Casale TB, et al. Allergic Rhinitis and its Impact on Asthma (ARIA) guidelines: 2010 revision. J Allergy Clin Immunol. 2010;126(3):466–76.
30. Jarvis D, Newson R, Lotvall J, Hastan D, Tomassen P, Keil T, et al. Asthma in adults and its association with chronic rhinosinusitis: the GA2LEN survey in Europe. Allergy. 2012;67(1):91–8.
31. Hirsch AG, Stewart WF, Sundaresan AS, Young AJ, Kennedy TL, Scott Greene J, et al. Nasal and sinus symptoms and chronic rhinosinusitis in a population-based sample. Allergy. 2017;72(2):274–81.
32. Schlosser RJ, Smith TL, Mace J, Soler ZM. Asthma quality of life and control after sinus surgery in patients with chronic rhinosinusitis. Allergy. 2017;72(3):483–91.
33. Chen Y, Dales R, Lin M. The epidemiology of chronic rhinosinusitis in Canadians. Laryngoscope. 2003;113(7):1199–205.
34. Hamilos DL. Chronic rhinosinusitis: epidemiology and medical management. J Allergy Clin Immunol. 2011;128(4):693–707; quiz 8-9.

Distinguishing Asthma from Comorbid Conditions in Older Adults

Joram S. Seggev

As discussed in the previous chapters, asthma is often underdiagnosed and undertreated in older adults. Asthma, allergic rhinitis, and sinusitis are common conditions in older adults and more prevalent in women than in men [1, 2]. Asthma is recognized less often in this population and is frequently undertreated. Cough is prevalent among older asthmatics [3–7]. Perception of dyspnea is markedly reduced [4]. While wheezing is still the most common complaint of asthma in the older asthmatic, the differential diagnosis is broad [3–7]. Because of multiple comorbidities in this population, particularly cardiovascular disease (CVD), symptoms are frequently ascribed to heart disease rather than asthma. COPD (chronic obstructive pulmonary disease) and asthma-COPD overlap syndrome (ACOS) need to be distinguished from asthma because of their prevalence and because they require different therapeutic approaches. Absence of acute reversibility on pulmonary function testing does not exclude asthma; normal diffusion capacity makes COPD less likely. By the same token, a normal level of B-type natriuretic peptide and a chest X-ray with no signs of congestion lessen the likelihood of heart failure. Common comorbidities that mimic or exacerbate asthma include rhinosinusitis, gastroesophageal reflux disease (GERD), and medications such as beta-blockers. Care needs to be taken not to confuse the following common causes of respiratory symptoms with asthma: heart failure, airway obstruction by functional or structural abnormalities, foreign bodies, tumors, and external compression or infiltration. A patient often suffers from more than one condition. Careful, comprehensive evaluation is necessary for proper management of the older adult with asthma.

Airway hyperreactivity may actually be more prevalent among older adults than in younger adults [3]. Because of the high prevalence of chronic diseases in older patients, many asthmatics suffer from more than one comorbid condition [3–7]. Comorbid conditions and medications may affect or mimic asthma as well as

J. S. Seggev (✉)
Internal Medicine, College of Medicine, Roseman University of Health Sciences, Las Vegas, NV, USA
e-mail: jseggev@roseman.edu

© Springer Nature Switzerland AG 2019
T. E. G. Epstein, S. M. Nyenhuis (eds.), *Treatment of Asthma in Older Adults*,
https://doi.org/10.1007/978-3-030-20554-6_4

complicate its management (see Tables 4.1 and 4.2) [3–10]. An Australian population survey of 37,000 adults aged 65 years and older found those with asthma had more comorbid diseases than those without asthma [11]. Dyspnea as a symptom of asthma is less prevalent among older adult asthmatics [4]. A brief review of dyspnea with representative clinical vignettes was published in 2013 [12].

Table 4.1 The major differential diagnosis of asthma in older adults

Diagnosis	Major features	Comments and suggestions
COPD/ACOS	See Table 4.3 for details	
Upper airway cough syndrome (UACS)		
Rhinitis, allergic and non-allergic	Prevalent atrophic and gustatory rhinitis; typical allergic symptoms may be reduced; cough; airway hyperreactivity	Allergy testing if indicated; therapeutic trial Rhinoscopy; sinus CT
Rhinosinusitis	Halitosis; irritant cough and throat clearing prominent; nasal polyps; recurrent sinusitis	Rhinoscopy; sinus CT
Congestive heart failure	Exertional and/or nighttime dyspnea; wheezing with pulmonary congestion	Appropriate history and physical examination; B-natriuretic peptide (BNP); chest X-ray (CXR); ECG
Pulmonary emboli	Sudden severe dyspnea and chest tightness; wheezing $\leq 10\%$; hemoptysis 6%	Some asymptomatic; D-dimer; lower extremities venous Doppler; pulmonary CT angiography
Gastroesophageal reflux disease (GERD)	Nighttime (or recumbent) cough and occasional wheeze; throat clearing	24-hour pH monitoring; improvement with trial of anti-reflux measures and proton pump inhibitors
Chronic aspiration	Cough and sputum production major and wheeze minor; bedridden and debilitated patients	May develop atelectasis, recurrent pneumonia; CXR; evaluation of swallowing
Airway obstruction, mechanical and functional		
Tumors, laryngeal and tracheal and stenosis, from intubation/radiation	Hoarseness; inspiratory wheeze and/or stridor; dyspnea, mainly inspiratory	Fixed obstruction on flow/volume curves; endoscopy; CXR indicated to exclude intra-thoracic causes
Bronchial tumors and foreign bodies	Cough, localized wheeze; dyspnea variable; obstructive pneumonia may occur	CXR; chest CT; bronchoscopy
External pressure or infiltration by tumors	Localized wheeze and dyspnea; other symptoms variable	CXR; chest CT
Endobronchial granulomata, TB and non-infectious (e.g., sarcoidosis)	Irritant cough, usually dry, dyspnea, and wheeze variable	CXR; sputum studies; chest CT; bronchoscopy
Vocal cord dysfunction	Labored breathing; stridor prominent; wheeze variable	Blunted inspiratory flow/volume curve; laryngoscopy May be functional or associated with asthma and GERD
Hyperventilation syndromes	Hyperventilation and labored breathing; may have stridor	Mostly functional, but can occur along with asthma and secondary to central nervous system disorders

Table 4.2 Rare causes of and medications causing asthma or asthma-like symptoms

Diagnosis	Major feature(s)	Comments and suggestions
Allergic bronchopulmonary aspergillosis (ABPA)	Steroid-dependent asthma in most; central bronchiectasis; *Aspergillus* in sputum	Specific and high total IgE; specific IgG; positive skin tests; chest CT
Bronchiectasis	Cough; purulent, copious sputum	CXR; chest CT diagnostic
Cystic fibrosis	Recurrent bronchitis, purulent sputum; GI symptoms; symptoms of variable intensity	Possible family history; sweat test Definitive – genetic testing
Carcinoid (endobronchial)	Usually presents as obstructive tumor, may cause localized persistent wheeze	CXR, chest CT; usually does not cause the carcinoid syndrome
EGPA (Churg-Strauss syndrome)	Vasculitis with extravascular eosinophils; severe asthma, usually preceding; rhinosinusitis; variable pulmonary infiltrates	Eosinophilia >10^3/mm³; elevated CRP possibly better than ESR (only ~60%); ANCA 40–60% of patients; sinus and chest CT
Systemic mastocytosis	Lung least affected organ; very rare; wheeze and cough reported	For screening – serum tryptase
Medications		
Angiotensin-converting enzyme inhibitors (ACEI)	Cough in 10% of patients; rare wheezing; may also develop angioedema with frequent involvement of head and neck	Cough may subside only after 3 weeks of stopping treatment; most patients can tolerate an ARB
ARB antagonists	At least 1% of patients may develop cough	Substitute the medication to another class
Non-selective beta-blockers, systemic and ophthalmic	Wheezing, airway hyperirritability, increased use of $\beta 2$ agonists, dyspnea	Substitute the medication; most patients can tolerate a $\beta 1$-selective blocker
Aspirin and NSAID	Acute asthma exacerbation or worsening of otherwise stable asthma, frequently along with sinusitis or nasal polyps	Ideally stop the medication; substitute acetaminophen, non-aspirin salicylates, or celecoxib. Desensitize in selected cases
Iodinated radio-contrast materials	Anaphylactoid reactions, angioedema and acute asthma	May occur even in spite of proper premedication and the use of non-ionized contrast media
Corticosteroids	Very rare; acute asthma and anaphylactoid reactions	Occurred mainly with prednisolone and methylprednisolone and less with hydrocortisone

ANCA anti-neutrophil cytoplasmic antibody, *ARB* angiotensin receptor-binding antagonist, *CRP* C-reactive protein, *CT* computerized tomography, *CXR* chest X-ray, *EGPA* eosinophilic granulomatosis with polyangiitis, *ESR* erythrocyte sedimentation rate, *NSAID* nonsteroidal anti-inflammatory agents

The Role of Allergic Rhinitis and Sinusitis

"Common wisdom" suggests that allergic rhinosinusitis is rare in older asthmatics. Atopy may still be significant in these patients. In the 2012 National Health Interview Survey (NHIS) survey, the prevalence of allergic rhinitis and sinusitis was 7.9% and 13.9% among people aged 65–74 years old, respectively, with women affected more than men. Among people age 75 years and older, the corresponding numbers were 5.4% and 9.9% [1]. A study that was based on the 2005–2006 National Health and Nutrition Examination Survey (NHANES) found no significant difference in atopy between younger asthmatics and those over age 55, although older adults were more likely to be sensitized to house dust mite and pets [13]. Another study confirmed the presence of allergy to indoor allergens in patients over 60 years of age [14]. Two small studies with older adult patients (mean age = 61 years), reported together, suggested that sensitization to cat and house dust mite was more likely to be associated with the development of airway hyperreactivity [15]. In another study of 66 asthmatics with a mean age of 69 years, 21 patients were sensitized to house dust mite. These patients had a lower FEV_1, incomplete response to albuterol, and greater hyperinflation than non-sensitized patients [16]. In a recent study in Brazil of 243 asthmatics (mean age 70.5 +/− 6.9 years), 71% of whom were severe, atopy was detected in 62.9% of the patients. House dust mite sensitivity was detected in 57.4% [17]. In a study of sinusitis, the severity of inflammation on CT scanning of the sinuses was greater among older than younger allergic patients. In that study, 45% (10/22) had asthma as well [18]. In the European GA^2LEN study, there was a strong association of asthma with chronic rhinosinusitis (CRS) at all ages [19]. The association with asthma was stronger in those reporting both CRS and allergic rhinitis. CRS in the absence of nasal allergies was positively associated with late-onset asthma [19]. In a study of severe asthmatics, those with severe CRS on CT scans had higher peripheral blood and sputum eosinophils, higher exhaled nitric oxide levels, lower diffusion capacity, and higher functional residual capacity (FRC). The latter findings correlated more with patients suffering from adult-onset asthma [20]. On the other hand, rhinosinusitis is a major cause of chronic cough, currently termed upper airway cough syndrome. It is important to distinguish upper airway cough syndrome from asthma and gastroesophageal reflux disease (GERD)-induced cough [21].

Asthma, Chronic Obstructive Pulmonary Disease (COPD), and Asthma-COPD Overlap Syndrome (ACOS)

The current definition of asthma maintains that it is a heterogeneous disease, usually associated with chronic airway inflammation. Symptoms include intermittent wheezing, cough and dyspnea, as well as variable airway obstruction [22]. As is the case with asthma in younger patients, the disease is variable in its symptomatology among older patients, as well as in the same patient. The perception of the typical asthma symptoms is generally decreased in older adults with asthma [3–5, 7]. Wheezing in this population is associated with more significant airway obstruction than in younger patients [3]. On the other hand, not every wheeze suggests asthma; clinicians should be vigilant not to miss other diseases that can also cause wheezing such as COPD, intra-bronchial obstruction, heart failure, and pulmonary embolism. For more details, see below and Tables 4.1 and 4.2 [3–7, 12]. COPD is characterized by persistent respiratory symptoms and airway obstruction, due to changes in the airways and/or alveoli, and is usually caused by exposure to tobacco smoke (most common) and other noxious particles or gases [23]. ACOS patients have features of both asthma and COPD. These patients may have suffered from allergy or "typical" asthma symptoms in childhood, or may have current allergy symptoms and elevated IgE. They may also be "non-atopic" asthmatics, smoking asthmatics, or non-smoking asthmatics with persistent airway obstruction. Smoking may be a factor in a significant number of these patients [22–25]. Patients with ACOS suffer more exacerbations of their disease and a more rapid decline of lung function than patients with asthma alone [24, 25]. The main distinguishing features between asthma, COPD, and ACOS are presented in Table 4.3. Helpful features may

Table 4.3 Comparison of asthma, ACOS, and COPD

Factor	Asthma	ACOS	COPD
Onset	Usually before age 20, may occur at any age	Usually at age ≥ 40; may have had symptoms when young	Age ≥ 40 in most cases
Typical symptoms	Great variability; usual asthma triggers causing symptoms	Chronic symptoms with better and worse days, dyspnea on exercise	Initially minimal, increasing dyspnea, variable cough, and sputum production
Past and family history	Family and/or personal history of atopy and asthma	Similar to asthma patients, but may also have smoked and/or been exposed to irritants	Tobacco smoke predominant and/or exposure to irritants
Typical natural history	Variable response to proper therapy, from complete to partial	Symptomatic improvement with treatment; often progressive, chronic treatment required Significant comorbidities	Slow progressive worsening in spite of treatment Significant comorbidities
Pulmonary function tests (PFT) Bronchodilator (BD) Diffusion capacity (DLco)	Evidence of airway hyperreactivity, good response to inhaled BD Normal to high DLco except when acute	Constant airway obstruction, significant but incomplete reversibility to inhaled BD DLco normal or reduced	May have some reversibility to inhaled BD, but FEV_1/FVC < 70% DLco reduced
Radiology	Chest X-ray usually normal; CT scan may be abnormal	Hyperinflation common CT scan invariably abnormal	Hyperinflation nearly universal; CT scan abnormal
Airway cytology	Eosinophils and/or neutrophils	Eosinophils and/or neutrophils	Mainly neutrophils; eosinophils in some patients; lymphocytes in airways
Exhaled nitric oxide (FE_{NO})	Levels elevated in atopic and eosinophilic asthma (see text)	Levels may range from low to increased	FE_{NO} levels usually low, may be elevated if eosinophils present
Approach to treatment	Treat as asthma per NAEPP/GINA guidelines	Initially try to treat as asthma; consider anti-cholinergic agents early	Per GOLD guidelines

NAEPP National Asthma Education and Prevention Program, *GINA* Global Initiative for Asthma, *GOLD* Global Initiative for Chronic Obstructive Lung Disease
Adapted from Refs. [22–24, 26–31]

be physiological; in ACOS, evidence of airway obstruction is always present with an FEV_1/FVC <70% (ratio of forced expiratory volume to forced vital capacity), possible hyperinflation, and normal/decreased diffusion capacity. In many cases, there is significant reversibility of FEV_1 to inhaled bronchodilator of ≥15% and ≥400 mL, or at least a response of ≥12% and ≥200 mL, on ≥2 occasions [24, 25]. In COPD, evidence of airway obstruction is always present with an FEV_1/FVC <70% and hyperinflation and may have a decreased diffusion capacity. Still, many COPD patients may have significant reversibility at times, particularly those with sputum eosinophilia. "Pure" asthmatics will have either a normal or increased diffusion capacity unless they suffer from acute or significant airway obstruction [24–26, 30]. Another feature is exhaled nitric oxide (Fe_{NO}) levels. Fe_{NO} concentration in older adults is higher than in younger adults [27]. In allergic asthma, particularly if poorly controlled, Fe_{NO} levels will be elevated. However, a study of 30 older adult asthmatics whose disease duration ranged from 2 to 70 years detected no correlation between Fe_{NO} levels and disease activity or spirometry [28]. In smokers and in patients with neutrophilic asthma, Fe_{NO} levels will be lower. COPD patients typically have low Fe_{NO} levels, except those with sputum eosinophilia. FE_{NO} levels in COPD patients with sputum eosinophilia are usually lower than in eosinophilic asthma [27]. In ACOS patients, Fe_{NO} levels are in between what is seen in asthma and COPD patients, and the degree of atopy and smoking may impact levels [29]. Radiological features in older adults may be complicated by comorbidities. In their absence, chest X-rays (CXR) of asthmatic patients may be normal or show hyperinflation and airway thickening. Computed tomography of the chest (chest CT) may show abnormalities in quite a number of asthma patients, although it is not routinely indicated unless complications such as allergic bronchopulmonary aspergillosis (ABPA), bronchiectasis, or exclusion of another disease are suspected [31, 32]. In early COPD, CXR may be normal; later on, similar changes to asthma may be seen as well as air trapping, hyperlucency, and bullae. Chest CT is typically abnormal in COPD. Changes in ACOS will be intermediate, depending on the severity of the disease [31, 32]. A recent study of 180 older adults with asthma by Baptist et al. suggested 4 phenotypes of asthma ranging from the "typical" allergic asthma patient whose disease began at a young age to the most severe, whose pulmonary function, asthma control, and quality of life were markedly reduced [32]. The latter group would be the one to consider whether those patients suffer from "true" asthma or from COPD or ACOS. The main significance of the diagnosis is in the management of those patients. Asthma patients should be treated according to current guidelines [22]. Per the Global Initiative for Chronic Obstructive Lung Disease (GOLD) guidelines, patients with "pure" COPD should have inhaled corticosteroids added only if experiencing severe disease or suffering from multiple exacerbations [23]. A recent study of thousands of moderate and severe COPD patients suggested that treatment with a triple medication inhaler of long-acting beta-agonist agents (LABA), long-acting muscarinic agents (LAMA), and Inhaled CorticoSteroids (ICS) led to better spirometry and reduced exacerbations when compared with an inhaler containing only LABA and ICS [33]. ACOS patients, particularly those with significant asthma symptoms and/or allergic disease, should be treated like asthma patients and should not be treated with a LABA or LAMA therapy without an ICS. However, older patients may respond better to LAMA than LABA, possibly more so in patients with incomplete reversibility on pulmonary function testing [22–25].

Cardiovascular Diseases (CVD)

Hypertension affects 52.3% of people aged 65–74 years and 59.2% of those aged ≥75 years. Coronary artery disease (CAD) is estimated to affect 16.2% and 25.8% in those age groups, respectively [34]. The prevalence of both diseases increases the likelihood of a patient suffering from asthma and CVD or only from the latter. Furthermore, some studies suggested an increased prevalence of CVD in patients with asthma or allergic rhinitis [35, 36]. Both CVD and some of the medications used to treat them can worsen asthma or cause symptoms that mimic asthma [3, 37–40] (see below and Table 4.2). However, cardiac asthma, per se, is unrelated to bronchial asthma. The clinical symptoms of cardiac asthma are caused by pulmonary venous hypertension due to either systolic or diastolic heart failure [37, 38]. The list of diseases causing heart failure is very long, but the most common are CAD and hypertensive cardiomyopathy [37, 38]. The main cause of dyspnea in the cardiac patient is pulmonary venous congestion due to the larger venous return when recumbent or during exercise. Lung function can be significantly affected by the excess water associated with venous congestion and later fluid retention [37–39, 41]. Total lung capacity may be reduced by interstitial edema, and having an enlarged heart and pleural effusions may further compress the lungs. Lung compliance will decrease, requiring increased respiratory effort that may lead to muscle fatigue [37–39, 42]. Resistance to airflow can be increased because of (1) reflex bronchoconstriction caused by the increased capillary hydrostatic pressure and edema; (2) compression of the bronchi by the stiff lung; and (3) bronchial obstruction from intra-luminal fluid and mucosal edema. These changes may cause wheezing [3, 37–39, 42]. The clinical picture of cardiac asthma depends on the patient's heart function. Patients at New York Heart Association (NYHA) class I (no symptoms) may have a perfectly normal physical examination; if those patients have asthma are well, their respiratory symptoms may be ascribed to their asthma. On the other hand, in patients with NYHA class IV (severe symptoms at rest, nearly bedridden), it may be very difficult clinically to determine whether their symptoms are due to asthma [37, 38].

"Classical" cardiac asthma has been described as late-night episodes of shortness of breath, cough, usually non-productive, and wheezing (paroxysmal nocturnal dyspnea, PND). Hemoptysis may occur. Sitting or standing up and sometimes opening a window will ameliorate the symptoms. Sleeping in a semi-recumbent position may help prevent the attacks [37, 38, 41]. Cardiac asthma does suggest advanced heart failure. The fact that some cardiac patients may be mistaken for having asthma has been known for nearly 200 years [42]. Still, physical examination during the day may or may not detect signs of heart failure. Cough may be present in both diseases. Physical activity causing shortness of breath, cough, and/or wheezing, with a good response to inhaled bronchodilators, suggests asthma. To muddy the waters even further, some "pure" cardiac patients may respond, at least partially, to beta-2 agonists [37–39, 41]. On physical examination, subtle findings, such as a S3 gallop, or overt findings, such as wet rales over both lungs, suggest left-sided heart failure [37–39]. The most helpful diagnostic tests for the detection of heart failure are the serum B-type natriuretic peptide (BNP) level and echocardiography. The latter can determine the size of the cardiac chambers, ejection fraction, valvular function, and the presence of pericardial effusion. CXR can be diagnostic, if positive for signs of left-sided heart failure (venous congestion to florid pulmonary edema, Kerley B lines, and/or an enlarged heart) [37–39]. BNP is one of three related hormones: (1) atrial NP (ANP), secreted by the atria, and (2 and 3) BNP and N-terminal proBNP (NT-proBNP), secreted by the atria and ventricles in response to increased volume or pressure [43, 44]. A normal (<100 pg/mL) level of BNP is incompatible with heart failure, while a BNP level of $\geq$400 pg/mL is highly suggestive of heart failure [37, 38, 43]. The use of BNP measurement in patients with asthma and/or COPD increases the diagnosis of heart failure by 20% [37, 38, 43–44]. Some severe COPD patients have elevated levels of BNP; BNP levels in those patients are significantly lower than in patients with heart failure. Stable COPD patients usually will have normal BNP and NT-proBNP levels [44]. Furthermore, BNP levels may be reduced by inhaled $\beta2$ agonists [44]. In summary, patients who complain of symptoms of "cardiac asthma" have no abnormalities on physical examination but have increased BNP and NT-proBNP and most likely suffer from heart failure. However, if a known cardiac patient who also suffers from asthma or COPD has normal BNP and NT-proBNP levels and has no signs of congestion on CXR, the likelihood of heart failure is slim [4, 37–39, 43, 44].

Pulmonary Emboli

The symptomatology of pulmonary emboli (PE) ranges from none to sudden death. PE is mentioned as a cause for wheezing in many reviews of asthma in older adults [3–7]. Episodic to sudden dyspnea and wheezing occur in a fraction of patients. In a series of 119 patients with documented pulmonary emboli, 10 (8%) developed wheezing. In the same series of patients, ages 71–80 years, a greater incidence of isolated dyspnea than pulmonary infarction was found. Younger and older patients had a similar incidence of both. There was no difference in the incidence of wheezing in the two groups. Hemoptysis occurred only with pulmonary infarction, and 14 of 119 (12%) had neither dyspnea nor tachypnea [45]. In another series of 154 patients with PE, 9.1% developed wheezing. Patients with previous cardiopulmonary disease seemed to be more likely to develop wheezing, but the difference did not reach significance [46]. A review of autopsies in Australia over a period of 10 years detected five cases of pulmonary emboli that were ascribed incorrectly to asthma before death [47]. A few series of PE patients in emergency rooms found no correlation between wheezing and PE. Two series found that patients with asthma and COPD presenting to an emergency room were less likely to have PE in spite of clinical suspicion [48, 49]. In patients who suffer from conditions that make PE more likely, such as recent surgery or prolonged inactivity, the presence of tachycardia, unexplained dyspnea, hemoptysis, and hypoxemia significantly increases the likelihood of PE [45, 46, 48, 49]. Testing for D-dimer, a breakdown product of fibrin, may be helpful. However, the values of normal levels of this test in younger patients have to be adjusted for patients older than 50 years [50].

Gastroesophageal Reflux Disease (GERD)

The reflux of gastric contents to the esophagus is more common among asthma patients than in healthy people [51, 52]. It seems that the prevalence of reflux does not differ between asymptomatic and symptomatic GERD patients with asthma; the asymptomatic patients actually have more acid reflux than the symptomatic patients [52]. Some studies have suggested that the pressure of the lower esophageal sphincter (LES) is reduced in asthma patients [52, 53]. Also, theophylline and beta-2 agonists can cause relaxation of the LES [52, 53]. Older adults may have different GERD symptoms than the typical symptoms found in younger patients. They are more likely to manifest anorexia, weight loss, anemia, vomiting, and dysphagia. The prevalence of severe esophagitis, larger hiatus hernia, gastric changes, and the use of NSAIDs also significantly increases with age [54]. Several studies have shown a correlation between GERD and rhinitis and cough and even cough-variant asthma [51, 55, 56, 70]. GERD has also been associated with cough and wheeze, although not necessarily with asthma; still, GERD may worsen asthma symptoms. GERD also has been associated with reduced quality of life in older adults with asthma [57–59]. One study actually found lower asthma exacerbation rates in older patients with GERD [60]. The available data on the effect of treating GERD on asthma are conflicting. Several reviews and studies suggest that the management of GERD leads, at the most, to symptomatic improvement in asthma and minor, if any, improvement in lung function or bronchial hyperactivity [51, 61–65]. Still, sub-populations may benefit from aggressive treatment, but are not well defined [61, 62]. A meta-analysis published in 1999 found that spirometry improved in only 27% of 417 asthmatics following fundoplication, whereas other symptoms improved in the majority of the patients [64]. A 2013 Finnish study of 69 patients, 12 of whom had asthma, addressed the effect of esomeprazole 40 mg BID or gastric fundoplication on the dose-response curve to a methacholine challenge, exhaled nitric oxide, and FEV_1. There was no improvement in any of these parameters. Cough and dyspnea improved with esomeprazole treatment and even more so after fundoplication. Among the patients with asthma, there was an improvement in the St. George Respiratory Questionnaire (SGRQ) scores as well [65]. Even a study that reported marked improvement in rhinitis, asthma, and GERD symptoms following endoscopic Stretta radiofrequency treatment to the lower esophagus and fundoplication refrained from reporting post-operative spirometry results; only pre-operative were reported, showing moderate airway obstruction [57]. While an asthma patient with symptomatic GERD has to be treated to reduce GERD symptoms, whether that treatment is going to improve asthma symptoms as well is still not quite settled. There is insufficient evidence to recommend routine administration of proton pump inhibitors in asthma [51, 61–63].

The relationship between GERD, obesity, and obstructive sleep apnea (OSA) is complicated [61, 66]. The latter two have also been associated with poor asthma control [61, 66–68]. However, obesity may be associated with wheezing and cough independent of asthma [61, 68, 69]. Furthermore, obese asthma patients whose disease began after age 12 have been shown to have milder, mainly neutrophilic, and non-atopic disease than obese asthma patients whose disease started at a younger age [69]. Severe asthma patients with a long history of disease tend to suffer from OSA [66–68]; asthma patients may develop OSA at higher rates than those without asthma [70]. A large Australian survey suggested that GERD caused respiratory symptoms directly, independent of BMI, risk of OSA, or airway hyperreactivity [71]. In summary, weight loss may help GERD, asthma, and OSA; patients with OSA still need to be treated for it. Patients should be screened for OSA and GERD and treated appropriately; obesity has to be addressed as well.

Mechanical Airway Obstruction (See Also Table 4.2) and Aspiration

Upper airway obstruction can be due to laryngeal, tracheal, and bronchial obstruction as well as factors external to the airways [3–7, 75, 76]. A plethora of causes of laryngeal obstruction exist. Common causes include: iatrogenic such as from thyroid or parathyroid surgery or damage to the recurrent laryngeal nerve; tumors of the larynx and of the thyroid and parathyroid; and idiopathic [72–75]. Glottic damage from anesthesia is not uncommon either [72, 73]. Even unilateral vocal cord palsy is associated with dyspnea [74]. The most common nonmalignant causes of tracheal and bronchial obstruction include granulation tissue resulting from endotracheal/tracheostomy tubes, foreign bodies, and tracheal or bronchomalacia. The main malignant tumors that can cause obstruction include bronchogenic, esophageal, and thyroid carcinoma [75]. Primary malignant tracheal tumors are rare [75]. An inspiratory wheeze or stridor is common along with attenuation or flattening of the inspiratory flow/volume curve. This occurs usually in obstruction proximal to the sternal notch [3, 72, 75]. Lower tracheal and bronchial obstruction will usually lead to signs of cough, expiratory wheezing, and changes in the expiratory loop of the flow/volume curve. With fixed obstruction, whether intra- or extra-thoracic, the whole flow/volume curve will be affected [3, 72, 75]. At that point, reduced air flow, and inspiratory and expiratory wheezing may be present. On the other hand, wheezes may be localized to an area of the chest, depending on the location of the obstruction. Of the causes of intra-bronchial obstruction, the most common is bronchogenic carcinoma, which is also a major cause of mortality in the older adults [75, 76]. Other causes include thoracic tumors infiltrating or compressing the airways and aortic aneurysms [75]. Less frequent or rare causes include foreign bodies that can cause complete occlusion by themselves or due to associated swelling and inflammation [75, 77–79]; carcinoid tumor [77, 79]; intra-bronchial tuberculosis and actinomycosis [75, 80, 81]; non-infectious mucosal granulomata, e.g., sarcoid [77, 82]; intra-bronchial metastases of breast, colon, and kidney cancer and lymphomata [77, 83]; post-irradiation stenosis [84]; aortic aneurysms [3, 75]; and dilated pulmonary artery [85].

Aspiration may result in airway obstruction. It occurs more frequently into the right lung because of the position of the right main bronchus [77]. Risk factors for aspiration include diminished consciousness and neuromuscular disorders affecting swallowing such as cerebrovascular accidents and degenerative diseases which impact older adults more frequently [79, 86]. A history of sudden violent cough with or without wheezing followed by persistent mild symptoms suggests acute aspiration. As mentioned earlier, aspiration can cause airway obstruction mechanically or with the addition of mucosal swelling and inflammation. Chronic aspiration may be associated with minor symptoms [79, 86].

Localized wheezing is always a "red flag" suggesting a localized lesion as opposed to the diffuse wheezing of asthma. Besides history and physical examination, spirometry and a CXR are a must for any older patient with new-onset cough, wheeze, and dyspnea [3–7, 75]. Further testing would depend on the clinical suspicion raised by the initial evaluation.

Medications (Also See Table 4.2)

Angiotensin-converting enzyme inhibitors (ACEI) cause cough in up to 20% of patients; they rarely cause wheezing [87–90]. Due to the high prevalence of heart disease and hypertension in older adults, ACEIs are a common culprit for cough. Angiotensin receptor-binding antagonists (ARBs) are less likely to cause cough and can be tolerated by most patients [90]. Non-selective beta-blockers are another common cause for wheezing, cough, and occasional dyspnea due to their use in heart disease and hypertension. Topical administration, such as timolol, for glaucoma may be the culprit and has even caused death [91, 92]. Directed questioning and asking patients to bring all their medications for appointments may be helpful. Beta-1 selective blockers will be tolerated by most asthma patients, but the lowest possible dose should be used [91]. Aspirin-exacerbated respiratory disease (AERD) [93] may lead to asthma flares because of (1) the high prevalence of CAD requiring frequent or chronic administration of low-dose aspirin [40] and (2) the frequent use of NSAIDs in the older adult population, making them a significant cause of emergency room visits [94]. Many patients with AERD can be successfully desensitized, if necessary [95]. Iodinated radio-contrast media (RCM) can cause bronchospasm at any age. RCM are also used during cardiac catheterizations, making them a real problem. Not every patient can be protected from a reaction even with proper premedication and the use of non-ionized RCM [96, 97]. A very rare cause of asthma symptoms is systemic corticosteroids (CS). In a Swiss survey, of 13 patients with systemic hypersensitivity reactions, three developed an acute asthma attack [98]. In a meta-analysis of reactions to CS in 106 patients, only 6 patients developed bronchospasm to intravenous CS (3 to methylprednisolone and 3 to prednisolone). Sixty-seven patients developed anaphylaxis to a variety of CS. However, the 2 medications mentioned above led to 41 reactions (of 120 reactions, meaning that some patients had more than 1 reaction) [99].

Vocal Cord Dysfunction (VCD) and Hyperventilation Syndromes

Obstruction due to vocal cord dysfunction manifests as difficulty in inhalation, often with stridor, due to closure of the vocal cords during inspiration. It can present as a functional disorder, mainly in younger patients. It can be triggered by exercise and may be associated with anxiety and other psychiatric disorders. Distraction can be effective as acute treatment, but severe attacks may require helium inhalation. Long-term treatment is speech therapy [72, 100, 101]. VCD can be confused with severe asthma; it can occur in up to 75% of asthmatics, which makes the diagnosis even harder. VCD can be associated with chronic irritation of the vocal cords by GERD, laryngopharyngeal reflux, rhinitis, or exposure to chemical or sensory irritants. Appropriate treatment and avoidance of triggers may significantly improve symptoms in such patients [72, 100, 101]. Symptoms associated with GERD may be different than in "pure" psychogenic VCD [100]. An abnormal inspiratory flow volume curve on spirometry is suggestive; during acute episodes, the expiratory wheezing and phase of the flow/volume curve may be abnormal as well. Flexible laryngoscopy showing adduction of the vocal cords during inspiration is diagnostic [72, 101].

Acute and chronic hyperventilation may also be confused with asthma. While psychiatric disease is well known to be associated with hyperventilation, patients may suffer from physical disease including asthma and pulmonary emboli as well as central nervous system disease [102, 103].

Rare causes: Allergic bronchopulmonary aspergillosis (ABPA) occurs in at least 2% of adults with asthma, although estimates vary greatly. Patients with cystic fibrosis have a higher prevalence. ABPA is an excessive hypersensitivity reaction to fungal, not just *Aspergillus fumigatus* antigens, occurring in sensitized patients. Symptoms of ABPA include typical asthma and allergic rhinitis, but also expectoration of tan or brown sputum plugs, and low-grade fever [104, 105]. One case report describes an older adult with ABPA presenting with chronic cough alone [105]. Patients may be asymptomatic until significant lung destruction has occurred. Early diagnosis is crucial. Criteria for the diagnosis include asthma, high IgE levels, positive skin tests to and/or specific IgE and IgG to the offending fungus, and central bronchiectasis. In the absence of bronchiectasis, ABPA is considered serologic. Severe asthmatics should be evaluated for ABPA [104, 105].

Bronchiectasis may be congenital or acquired. Symptoms that may be confused with asthma are: cough; thick sputum production; dyspnea; and wheezing if the mucus causes sufficient obstruction to air flow [106]. Bronchiectasis has been detected in mild asthma patients and in a significant number of severe asthma patients with and without ABPA [104, 106, 107]. Other causes include recurrent pulmonary infections, mainly associated with immune deficiency and persistent airway obstruction. The diagnosis is made by high-resolution CT scanning of the lung [30, 106].

Cystic fibrosis (CF) is the most common single-gene disease among Caucasian people. The median age of survival at this time is 44 years for females and 48 for males [108, 109]. Therefore, older patients suffering from the disease may be encountered. Atopic CF patients are more likely to develop ABPA as well. Severe asthma patients with rhinosinusitis and significant sputum production who respond poorly to treatment should be considered for evaluation for CF as well.

Carcinoid is the second most common bronchial tumor. The minority of carcinoids occur in the lung periphery [79]. The average age at diagnosis is 60 years, usually because of symptoms of bronchial obstruction. Up to a third of patients may be asymptomatic. Intra-bronchial carcinoid tumors represented 25.3% of 10,878 carcinoid tumors detected at any site. About 5% of patients develop the carcinoid syndrome caused by the release of serotonin and vasoactive peptides. The symptoms of the syndrome include systemic flushing, bronchospasm, diarrhea, disorientation, anxiety, tremor, hypotension, and tachycardia [81, 110].

Mastocytosis can rarely cause asthma symptoms [111, 112]. However, the respiratory tract is one of the least affected, along with the endocrine and renal systems [113]. The disease can occur at any age. Major symptoms include itching, flushing, abdominal pain, less often, diarrhea, nausea, and vomiting. Serum tryptase is a good measure for screening; a total tryptase level of >20 ng/mL is suggestive and requires further testing [113].

Eosinophilic granulomatosis with polyangiitis (EGPA), previously Churg-Strauss syndrome, is an eosinophilic necrotizing vasculitis. Although nearly all patients suffer from asthma prior to diagnosis [114–116], in the largest reported series of 383 patients with EGPA, the mean age was 50.3 ± 15.7 years, and 91.1% suffered from asthma [114]. The American College of Rheumatology for the disease requires at least four of six criteria: asthma, rhinosinusitis, mononeuritis multiplex, >10% blood eosinophils, intermittent pulmonary infiltrates, and extravascular eosinophils [114, 116]. Most patients will have an increased C-reactive protein, but only about 60% will have an increased erythrocyte sedimentation rate [114]. Antineutrophil cytoplasmic antibody is present in 40–60% of patients, depending on the specific report [114, 116]. Severe, steroid-dependent asthma with sinusitis and significant eosinophilia should at least raise the possibility of EGPA.

Summary

Asthma in older adults is not a rare disease. However, its symptoms may be more subtle than in younger adults. Furthermore, multiple co-existent diseases and their medications may mask the existence of asthma or worsen its symptoms. Treatment of the older adult is more difficult than the younger asthmatic because of comorbidities, reduced dexterity due to osteoarthritic changes, as well as cognitive decline. Taking a comprehensive history and performance of a physical examination, looking for symptoms and signs of asthma and allergy, and exclusion of other diseases are crucial. Pulmonary function testing looking for reversible obstruction and, if necessary, bronchial challenges are crucial. Lack of acute reversibility to bronchodilators does not rule out asthma. While drug therapy, in principle, is no different in this population, anti-cholinergic agents may be more effective than long-acting beta-2 agents. Comprehensive management of asthma and confounding comorbidities and potentially exacerbating medications is essential. Frail and/or asthmatics with decreased cognition may benefit from the involvement of family members, older adult day clubs, and/or visiting healthcare professionals.

References

1. Blackwell DL, Lucas JW, Clarke TC. Summary health statistics for U.S. adults: National Health Interview Survey, 2012. National Center for Health Statistics. Vital Health Stat. 2014;10(260):21. https://www.cdc.gov/nchs/data/series/sr_10/sr10_260.pd. Accessed Apr 2018.
2. Australian Institute of Health and Welfare 2018. Asthma Web report. Last updated 06/09/2017 v9.0. https://www.aihw.gov.au/reports/asthma-other-chronic-respiratory-conditions/asthma/data. Accessed 30 Mar 2018.
3. Ahmed T, Krieger BP, Wanner A. Differential diagnosis of asthma in the elderly. In: Barbee RA, Bloom JW, editors. Asthma in the elderly. New York: Marcel Dekker; 1997. p. 93–120.
4. Enright P. The diagnosis of asthma in older adults. Exp Lung Res. 2005;31(Suppl 1):15–21.
5. Mazen AA, Hassan T, Chotirmall SH. Advances in the diagnosis and management of asthma in older adults. Am J Med. 2014;127:370–8.
6. Hanania NA, King MJ, Braman SS, Saltoun C, Wise RA, Enright P, Falsey AR, et al. Asthma in the elderly: current understanding and future research needs – a report of a National Institute on Aging (NIA) workshop. J Allergy Clin Immunol. 2011;128(3 Suppl):S4–S24.
7. Gibson PG, McDonald VM, Marks GB. Asthma in older adults. Lancet. 2010;376:803–13.
8. Federal Interagency Forum on Aging-Related Statistics. Older Americans 2012: key indicators of well-being. Indicator 16, p. 27. Washington, DC: U.S. Government Printing Office; 2012.
9. Hsu J, Chen J, Mirabelli MC. Asthma morbidity, comorbidities, and modifiable factors among older adults. J Allergy Clin Immunol Pract. 2018;6:236–43.
10. Boulet LP. Influence of comorbid conditions on asthma. Eur Respir J. 2009;33:897–906.
11. Australian Centre for Asthma Monitoring 2008. Asthma in Australia 2008. AIHW Asthma Series no. 3. Cat. no. ACM 14. Canberra; 2008, p. 46–7.
12. Peters SP. When the chief complaint is (or should be) dyspnea in adults. J Allergy Clin Immunol Pract. 2013;1:129–36.
13. Busse PJ, Cohn RD, Salo PM, Zeldin DC. Characteristics of allergic sensitization among asthmatic adults older than 55 years: results from the National Health and Nutrition Examination Survey, 2005–2006. Ann Allergy Asthma Immunol. 2013;110:247–52.
14. Busse PJ, Lurslurchachai L, Sampson HA, Halm EA, Wisnivesky J. Perennial allergen-specific immunoglobulin E levels among inner-city elderly asthmatics. J Asthma. 2010;47(7):781–5.
15. Litonjua AA, Sparrow D, Weiss ST, O'Connor GT, Long AA, Ohman JL Jr. Sensitization to cat allergen is associated with asthma in older men and predicts new-onset airway hyperresponsiveness. The Normative Aging Study. Am J Respir Crit Care Med. 1997;156(1):23–7.
16. Rogers L, Cassino C, Berger KI, Goldring RM, Norman RG, Klugh T, et al. Asthma in the elderly: cockroach sensitization and severity of airway obstruction in elderly nonsmokers. Chest. 2002;122(5):1580–6.

17. Agondi RC, Andrade MC, Takejima P, Aun MV, Kalil J, Giavina-Bianchi P. Atopy is associated with age at asthma onset in elderly patients. J Allergy Clin Immunol Pract. 2017:S2213–198. (17)30874–7. https://doi.org/10.1016/j.jaip.2017.10.028.
18. Cho SH, Hong SJ, Han B, Lee SH, Suh L, Norton J, et al. Age-related differences in the pathogenesis of chronic rhinosinusitis. J Allergy Clin Immunol. 2012;129:858–60.
19. Jarvis D, Newson R, Lotvall J, Hastan D, Tomassen P, Keil T, et al. Asthma in adults and its association with chronic rhinosinusitis: the GA2LEN survey in Europe. Allergy. 2012;67:91–8.
20. ten Brinke A, Grootendorst DC, Schmidt JT, De Bruïne FT, van Buchem MA, Sterk PJ, et al. Chronic sinusitis in severe asthma is related to sputum eosinophilia. J Allergy Clin Immunol. 2002;109:621–6.
21. Pratter MR. Chronic upper airway cough syndrome secondary to rhinosinus diseases (previously referred to as postnasal drip syndrome): ACCP evidence-based clinical practice guidelines. Chest. 2006;129(Suppl):63S–71S.
22. Global Initiative for Asthma (GINA). Global strategy for asthma management and prevention; 2017:92. Available on line at www.ginasthma.com. Accessed Mar 2018.
23. Global Initiative for Chronic Obstructive Lung Disease (GOLD). Global strategy for the diagnosis, management and prevention of chronic obstructive pulmonary disease. Vancouver; 2017:6. Available from www.goldcopd.org/gold-reports
24. Putcha N, Wise RA. Asthma–chronic obstructive pulmonary disease overlap syndrome. Immunol Allergy Clin N Am. 2016;36:515–28.
25. Soler X, Ramsdell JW. Are asthma and COPD a continuum of the same disease? J Allergy Clin Immunol Pract. 2015;3:489–95.
26. Saydain G, Beck KC, Decker PA, Cowl CT, Scanlon PD. Clinical significance of elevated diffusing capacity. Chest. 2004;125:446–52.
27. Dweik RA, Boggs PB, Erzurum SC, Irvin CG, Leigh MW, Lundberg JO, et al. American Thoracic Society Committee on interpretation of exhaled nitric oxide levels (FENO) for clinical applications. Am J Respir Crit Care Med. 2011;184(5):602–15.
28. Columbo M, Wong B, Panettieri RA Jr, Rohr AS. Asthma in the elderly: the role of exhaled nitric oxide measurements. Respir Med. 2013;107(5):785–7.
29. Goto T, Camargo CA Jr, Hasegawa K. Fractional exhaled nitric oxide levels in asthma-COPD overlap syndrome: analysis of the National Health and Nutrition Examination Survey, 2007–2012. Int J Chron Obstruct Pulmon Dis. 2016;11:2149–55.
30. Richards JC, Lynch D, Koelsch T, Dyer D. Imaging of asthma. Immunol Allergy Clin North Am. 2016;36(3):529–45.
31. Han MK, Lazarus SC. COPD: diagnosis and clinical management. In: Broaddus VC, Mason RJ, Ernst JD, King TE, Lazarus SC, Murray JF, et al., editors. Murray & Nadel's textbook of respiratory medicine. 6th ed. Philadelphia: Saunders-Elsevier; 2016. p. 771.
32. Baptist AP, Hao W, Karamched KR, Kaur B, Carpenter L, PXK S. Distinct asthma phenotypes among older adults with asthma. J Allergy Clin Immunol Pract. 2018;6:244–9.
33. Lipson DA, Barnhart F, Brealey N, Brooks J, Criner GJ, Day NC, et al. Once-daily single-inhaler triple versus dual therapy in patients with COPD. N Engl J Med. 2018; https://doi.org/10.1056/NEJMoa1713901. [Epub ahead of print].
34. Blackwell DL, Lucas JW, Clarke TC. Summary health statistics for U.S. adults: National Health Interview Survey, 2012. National Center for Health Statistics. Vital Health Stat 2014;10(260):16. https://www.cdc.gov/nchs/data/series/sr_10/sr10_260.pd. Accessed Apr 2018.
35. Onufrak SJ, Abramson JL, Austin HD, Holguin F, McClellan WM, Vaccarino LV. Relation of adult-onset asthma to coronary heart disease and stroke. Am J Cardiol. 2008;101(9):1247–52.
36. Knoflach M, Kiechl S, Mayr A, Willeit J, Poewe W, Wick G. Allergic rhinitis, asthma, and atherosclerosis in the Bruneck and ARMY studies. Arch Intern Med. 2005;165(21):2521–6.
37. Tanabe T, Rozycki HJ, Kanoh S, Rubin BK. Cardiac asthma: new insights into an old disease. Expert Rev Respir Med. 2012;6(6):705–14.
38. Buckner K. Cardiac asthma. Immunol Allergy Clin N Am. 2013;33(1):35–44.

39. Hawkins NM, Petrie MC, Jhund PS, Chalmers GW, Dunn FG, McMurray JJ. Heart failure and chronic obstructive pulmonary disease: diagnostic pitfalls and epidemiology. Eur J Heart Fail. 2009;11(2):130–9.
40. Qato DM, Alexander GC, Conti RM, Johnson M, Schumm P, Lindau ST. Use of prescription and over-the-counter medications and dietary supplements among older adults in the United States. JAMA. 2008;300(24):2867–78.
41. Gehlbach BK, Geppert E. The pulmonary manifestations of left heart failure. Chest. 2004;125(2):669–82.
42. Fishman AP. Cardiac asthma – a fresh look at an old wheeze. N Engl J Med. 1989;320(20):1346–8.
43. Kim HN, Januzzi JL Jr. Natriuretic peptide testing in heart failure. Circulation. 2011;123(18):2015–9.
44. Calzetta L, Orlandi A, Page C, Rogliani P, Rinaldi B, Rosano G, et al. Brain natriuretic peptide: much more than a biomarker. Int J Cardiol. 2016;221:1031–8.
45. Stein PD, Henry JW. Clinical characteristics of patients with acute pulmonary embolism stratified according to their presenting syndromes. Chest. 1997;112(4):974–9.
46. Calvo-Romero JM, Pérez-Miranda M, Bureo-Dacal P. Wheezing in patients with acute pulmonary embolism with and without previous cardiopulmonary disease. Eur J Emerg Med. 2003;10(4):288–9.
47. Byard RW. All that wheezes is not asthma – alternative findings at autopsy. J Forensic Sci. 2011;56(1):252–5.
48. Kline JA, Kabrhel C. Emergency evaluation for pulmonary embolism, part 1: clinical factors that increase risk. J Emerg Med. 2015;48(6):771–80.
49. Kabrhel C, McAfee AT, Goldhaber SZ. The probability of pulmonary embolism is a function of the diagnoses considered most likely before testing. Acad Emerg Med. 2006;13(4):471–4.
50. Kline JA, Nelson RD, Jackson RE, Courtney DM. Criteria for the safe use of D-dimer testing in emergency department patients with suspected pulmonary embolism: a multicenter US study. Ann Emerg Med. 2002;39:144–52.
51. McCallister JW, Parsons JP, Mastronarde JG. The relationship between gastroesophageal reflux and asthma: an update. The relationship between gastroesophageal reflux and asthma: an update. Ther Adv Respir Dis. 2011;5(2):143–50.
52. Harding SM, Guzzo MR, Richter JE. The prevalence of gastroesophageal reflux in asthma patients without reflux symptoms. Am J Respir Crit Care Med. 2000;162(1):34–9.
53. Dua S, Mohan L. Lower esophageal sphincter pressures in patients of bronchial asthma and its correlation with spirometric parameters: a case-control study. J Asthma. 2016;53(3):289–94.
54. Pilotto A, Franceschi M, Leandro G, Scarcelli C, D'Ambrosio LP, Seripa D, et al. Clinical features of reflux esophagitis in older people: a study of 840 consecutive patients. J Am Geriatr Soc. 2006;54(10):1537–42.
55. Hellgren J, Olin AC, Torén K. Increased risk of rhinitis symptoms in subjects with gastro-esophageal reflux. Acta Otolaryngol. 2014;134(6):615–9.
56. Kanemitsu Y, Niimi A, Matsumoto H, Iwata T, Ito I, Oguma T, et al. Gastroesophageal dysmotility is associated with the impairment of cough-specific quality of life in patients with cough variant asthma. Allergol Int. 2016;65(3):320–6.
57. Hu Z, Wu J, Wang Z, Zhang Y, Liang W, Yan C. Outcome of Stretta radiofrequency and fundoplication for GERD-related severe asthmatic symptoms. Front Med. 2015;9(4):437–43.
58. Dąbrowska M, Grabczak EM, Arcimowicz M, Domeracka-Kołodziej A, Domagała-Kulawik J, Krenke R, et al. Causes of chronic cough in non-smoking patients. Adv Exp Med Biol. 2015;873:25–33.
59. Kannan JA, Bernstein DI, Bernstein CK, Ryan PH, Bernstein JA, Villareal MS, et al. Significant predictors of poor quality of life in older asthmatics. Ann Allergy Asthma Immunol. 2015;115(3):198–204.
60. Sumino K, O'Brian K, Bartle B, Au DH, Castro M, Lee TA. Coexisting chronic conditions associated with mortality and morbidity in adult patients with asthma. J Asthma. 2014;51(3):306–14.

61. Rogers L. Role of sleep apnea and gastroesophageal reflux in severe asthma. Immunol Allergy Clin N Am. 2016;36(3):461–71.
62. Gibson PG, Henry RL, Coughlan JL. Gastro-oesophageal reflux treatment for asthma in adults and children. Cochrane Database Syst Rev. 2003;2:CD001496.
63. Chan WW, Chiou E, Obstein KL, Tignor AS, Whitlock TL. The efficacy of proton pump inhibitors for the treatment of asthma in adults: a meta-analysis. Arch Intern Med. 2011;171(7):620–9.
64. Field SK, Gelfand GA, McFadden SD. The effects of antireflux surgery on asthmatics with gastroesophageal reflux. Chest. 1999;116(3):766–74.
65. Kiljander T, Rantanen T, Kellokumpu I, Kööbi T, Lammi L, Nieminen M, et al. Comparison of the effects of esomeprazole and fundoplication on airway responsiveness in patients with gastro-oesophageal reflux disease. Clin Respir J. 2013;7(3):281–7.
66. Diaz J, Farzan S. Clinical implications of the obese-asthma phenotypes. Immunol Allergy Clin North Am. 2014;34(4):739–51.
67. Teodorescu M, Polomis DA, Hall SV, Teodorescu MC, Gangnon RE, Peterson AG, et al. Association of obstructive sleep apnea risk with asthma control in adults. Chest. 2010;138(3):543–50.
68. Yigla M, Tov N, Solomonov A, Rubin AH, Harlev D. Difficult-to-control asthma and obstructive sleep apnea. J Asthma. 2003;40(8):865–71.
69. Holguin F, Bleecker ER, Busse WW, Calhoun WJ, Castro M, Erzurum SC, et al. Obesity and asthma: an association modified by age of asthma onset. J Allergy Clin Immunol. 2011;127(6):1486–93.
70. Teodorescu M, Barnet JH, Hagen EW, Palta M, Young TB, Peppard PE. Association between asthma and risk of developing obstructive sleep apnea. JAMA. 2015;313(2):156–64.
71. Mulrennan SA, Knuiman MW, Divitini ML, Cullen DJ, Hunter M, Hui J, et al. Gastro-oesophageal reflux and respiratory symptoms in Busselton adults: the effects of bodyweight and sleep apnoea. Intern Med J. 2012;42(7):772–9.
72. Morris MJ, Christopher KL. Diagnostic criteria for the classification of vocal cord dysfunction. Chest. 2010;138(5):1213–23.
73. Rosenthal LH, Benninger MS, Deeb RH. Vocal fold immobility: a longitudinal analysis of etiology over 20 years. Laryngoscope. 2007;117(10):1864–70.
74. Laccourreye O, Malinvaud D, Ménard M, Bonfils P. Unilateral laryngeal nerve paralysis in the adult: epidemiology, symptoms, physiopathology and treatment (French). Presse Med. 2014;43(4 Pt 1):348–52.
75. Ernst A, Feller-Kopman D, Becker HD, Mehta AC. Central airway obstruction. Am J Respir Crit Care Med. 2004;169(12):1278–97.
76. Siegel RL, Miller KD, Jemal A. Cancer statistics, 2015. CA Cancer J Clin. 2015;65(1):5–29.
77. Chen CH, Lai CL, Tsai TT, Lee YC, Perng RP. Foreign body aspiration into the lower airway in Chinese adults. Chest. 1997;112(1):129–33.
78. Lan RS. Non-asphyxiating tracheobronchial foreign bodies in adults. Eur Respir J. 1994;7(3):510–4.
79. Modlin IM, Lye KD, Kidd M. A 5-decade analysis of 13,715 carcinoid tumors. Cancer. 2003;97(4):934–59.
80. Lee JH, Chung HS. Bronchoscopic, radiologic and pulmonary function evaluation of endobronchial tuberculosis. Respirology. 2000;5(4):411–7.
81. Chouabe S, Perdu D, Deslée G, Milosevic D, Marque E, Lebargy F. Endobronchial actinomycosis associated with foreign body: four cases and a review of the literature. Chest. 2002;121(6):2069–72.
82. Polychronopoulos VS, Prakash UBS. Airway involvement in sarcoidosis. Chest. 2009;136(5):1371–80.
83. Froudarakis ME, Bouros D, Siafakas NM. Endoluminal metastases of the tracheobronchial tree: is there any way out? Chest. 2001;119(3):679–81.
84. Cho YC, Kim JH, Park JH, Shin JH, Ko HK, Song HY. Fluoroscopically guided balloon dilation for benign bronchial stricture occurring after radiotherapy in patients with lung cancer. Cardiovasc Intervent Radiol. 2014;37(3):750–5.

85. Dakkak W, Tonelli AR. Compression of adjacent anatomical structures by pulmonary artery dilation. Postgrad Med. 2016;128(5):451–9.
86. Feinberg MJ, Knebl J, Tully J, Segall L. Aspiration and the elderly. Dysphagia. 1990;5(2):61–71.
87. Semple PF. Putative mechanisms of cough after treatment with angiotensin converting enzyme inhibitors. J Hypertens Suppl. 1995;13(3):S17–21.
88. Kaufman J, Schmitt S, Barnard J, Busse W. Angiotensin-converting enzyme inhibitors in patients with bronchial responsiveness and asthma. Chest. 1992;101(4):922–5.
89. Semple PF, Herd GW. Cough and wheeze caused by inhibitors of angiotensin-converting enzyme. N Engl J Med. 1986;314(1):61.
90. Lacourcière Y, Brunner H, Irwin R, Karlberg BE, Ramsay LE, Snavely DB, et al. Effects of modulators of the renin-angiotensin-aldosterone system on cough. Losartan cough study group. J Hypertens. 1994;12(12):1387–93.
91. Morales DR, Jackson C, Lipworth BJ, Donnan PT, Guthrie B. Adverse respiratory effect of acute β-blocker exposure in asthma: a systematic review and meta-analysis of randomized controlled trials. Chest. 2014;145(4):779–86.
92. Morales DR, Dreischulte T, Lipworth BJ, Donnan PT, Jackson C, Guthrie B. Respiratory effect of beta-blocker eye drops in asthma: population-based study and meta-analysis of clinical trials. Br J Clin Pharmacol. 2016;82(3):814–22.
93. Bochenek G, Niżankowska-Mogilnicka E. Aspirin-exacerbated respiratory disease: clinical disease and diagnosis. Immunol Allergy Clin N Am. 2013;33(2):147–61.
94. Budnitz DS, Pollock DA, Weidenbach KN, Mendelsohn AB, Schroeder TJ, Annest JL. National surveillance of emergency department visits for outpatient adverse drug events. JAMA. 2006;296(15):1851–7.
95. Woessner KM, Simon RA. Cardiovascular prophylaxis and aspirin "allergy". Immunol Allergy Clin North Am. 2013;33(2):263–74.
96. Morcos SK. Review article: effects of radiographic contrast media on the lung. Br J Radiol. 2003;76(905):290–5.
97. Liccardi G, Salzillo A, De Blasio F, D'Amato G. Control of asthma for reducing the risk of bronchospasm in asthmatics undergoing general anesthesia and/or intravascular administration of radiographic contrast media. Curr Med Res Opin. 2009;25(7):1621–30.
98. Caduff C, Reinhart WH, Hartmann K, Kuhn M. Immediate hypersensitivity reactions to parenteral glucocorticoids? Analysis of 14 cases [German]. Schweiz Med Wochenschr. 2000;130(26):977–83.
99. Patel A, Bahna SL. Immediate hypersensitivity reactions to corticosteroids. Ann Allergy Asthma Immunol. 2015;115(3):178–82.
100. Parsons JP, Benninger C, Hawley MP, Philips G, Forrest LA, Mastronarde JG. Vocal cord dysfunction: beyond severe asthma. Respir Med. 2010;104(4):504–9.
101. Ibrahim WH1, Gheriani HA, Almohamed AA, Raza T. Paradoxical vocal cord motion disorder: past, present and future. Postgrad Med J. 2007;83(977):164–172.
102. Bass C, Gardner WN. Respiratory and psychiatric abnormalities in chronic symptomatic hyperventilation. Br Med J (Clin Res Ed). 1985;290(6479):1387–90.
103. Brodtkorb E, Gimse R, Antonaci F, Ellertsen B, Sand T, Sulg I, et al. Hyperventilation syndrome: clinical, ventilatory, and personality characteristics as observed in neurological practice. Acta Neurol Scand. 1990;81(4):307–13.
104. Douglass JA, Sandrini A, Holgate ST, O'Hehir RE. Allergic bronchopulmonary aspergillosis. In: Adkinson NF, Bochner BS, Burks AW, Busse WW, Holgate ST, Lemanske RF, et al., editors. Middleton's allergy principles and practice. 8th ed. Philadelphia: Saunders-Elsevier; 2014. p. 1000–7.
105. Roth R, Schatz M. Allergic bronchopulmonary aspergillosis presenting as chronic cough in an elderly woman without previously documented asthma. Perm J. 2013;17(2):e103–8. https://doi.org/10.7812/TPP/12-051. (on-line only).
106. Truong T. The overlap of bronchiectasis and immunodeficiency with asthma. Immunol Allergy Clin North Am. 2013;33(1):61–78.

107. Coman I, Pola-Bibián B, Barranco P, Vila-Nadal G, Dominguez-Ortega J, Romero D, et al. Bronchiectasis in severe asthma: clinical features and outcomes. Ann Allergy Asthma Immunol. 2018;120(4):409–13.
108. Keogh RH, Stanojevic S. A guide to interpreting estimated median age of survival in cystic fibrosis patient registry reports. J Cyst Fibros. 2018;17(2):213–7.
109. Elborn JS. Cystic fibrosis. Lancet. 2016;388(10059):2519–31.
110. McIntire M, Shah ND, Kim AW, Gattuso P, Liptay MJ. Cytologic imprints of giant atypical bronchopulmonary carcinoid tumor of the lung with extensive oncocytic component. Diagn Cytopathol. 2008;36(12):887–90.
111. Boulet LP. Diagnosis of asthma in adults. In: Reference 104, p. 900.
112. Metcalfe DD. Mastocytosis. In: Adkinson NF, Bochner BS, Busse WW, Holgate ST, Lemanske RF, FER S, editors. Middleton's allergy principles and practice. 7th ed. Philadelphia: Saunders-Elsevier; 2009. p. 1053, Table 60.1.
113. Metcalfe DD. Mastocytosis. In: Reference 104, p. 1226.
114. Comarmond C, Pagnoux C, Khellaf M, Cordier JF, Hamidou M, Viallard JF, et al. Eosinophilic granulomatosis with polyangiitis (Churg-Strauss): clinical characteristics and long-term follow-up of the 383 patients enrolled in the French Vasculitis Study cohort. Arthritis Rheum. 2013;65:270–81.
115. Silva CI, Müller NL, Fujimoto K, Johkoh T, Ajzen SA, Churg A. Churg-Strauss syndrome: high resolution CT and pathologic findings. J Thorac Imaging. 2005;20(2):74–80.
116. King TE. Clinical features and diagnosis of eosinophilic granulomatosis with polyangiitis (Churg-Strauss). Up To Date 2018; literature review current through: Dec 2018: Topic 4347, Version 22.0.

Recent Barriers to Effective Treatment of Asthma in Older Adults and Strategies to Address Them

5

Alan P. Baptist

Introduction

In this chapter, we will discuss some of the unique challenges that older adults face when it comes to optimal medical care. Rather than focusing on specific pharmacologic therapies (which will be discussed in other chapters), we will address issues that clinicians and care providers infrequently consider but can have a major impact on patient outcomes and satisfaction. These issues include items such as medical comorbidities, depression, obesity, menopause, hormone replacement therapy, care giver roles, complementary and alternative therapies, perception of breathlessness, and financial concerns.

Comorbidities

In recent years, there has been a significant increase in the literature demonstrating the effect of comorbidities on asthma management and control. A 2016 meta-analysis of 11 studies involving 460,000 patients found that asthma patients were more likely to have cardiovascular disease (odds ratio (OR) = 1.9), obesity (OR = 1.51), gut or urinary comorbidities (OR = 1.62), and hypertension (OR = 1.91) compared to those without asthma (p <0.0001 for all comparisons listed) [1]. The National Health and Nutrition Examination Survey (NHANES) found that adult asthma patients with comorbidities were more likely to have asthma symptoms, activity limitations, and emergency department visits for asthma compared to asthma patients without comorbidities [2]. Data specifically looking at adults ≥65 years has confirmed that in this age group, comorbidities are directly related to

A. P. Baptist (✉)
Division of Allergy and Clinical Immunology, Department of Internal Medicine, University of Michigan, Ann Arbor, MI, USA
e-mail: abaptist@med.umich.edu

© Springer Nature Switzerland AG 2019
T. E. G. Epstein, S. M. Nyenhuis (eds.), *Treatment of Asthma in Older Adults*,
https://doi.org/10.1007/978-3-030-20554-6_5

asthma hospitalizations and emergency department visits [3]. As people age, the number of medical conditions and medications to manage these conditions increase. Therefore, the negative impact of comorbidities and asthma management has a greater impact on older adults.

In older adults, comorbidities can impact asthma management in a number of ways. There can be interactions between conditions, similar symptom presentation of asthma and comorbidities, decreased adherence with multiple medications, and conflicting recommendations on care from numerous specialists [4]. In a qualitative study, older adults with asthma and cardiac disease describe having been instructed by their physician to try medications for both conditions simultaneously and/or sequentially during episodes of dyspnea [5]. Additionally, in patients with multiple comorbidities, asthma may take a "backseat" during a primary care office visit and be suboptimally addressed.

To improve the care of older adults with asthma, clinicians should identify, acknowledge, and address comorbidities where appropriate. A study by Tay et al. found that asthma outcomes improved when asthma specialists identified and subsequently treated or referred patients for specific comorbidities (e.g., GERD, sleep apnea, obesity) [6]. With improved control, it may be possible for the older adult to reduce the burden of other conditions such as cardiac disease, diabetes, and obesity.

Treatment of comorbid allergic rhinitis with nasal corticosteroids is a relatively safe approach in older adults and may be an option to improve asthma control without stepping up controller therapy [7]. Subcutaneous allergen immunotherapy improves allergic rhinitis in older patients and is reasonable to consider at any group, although risks including anaphylaxis and the use of epinephrine in patients with significant cardiac disease must be considered [8]. Sublingual immunotherapy has a lower incidence of serious adverse effects and may be an attractive alternative in older adults, though currently most formulations are approved only to the age 65. Subcutaneous or sublingual immunotherapy should not be initiated in patients whose asthma is poorly controlled [9].

Depression

While depression is an asthma comorbidity, it deserves additional mention due to recent literature showing its negative effects on older adults with asthma. Depression is relatively common in adults above the age of 65, affecting up to 20% of older adults in Western countries [10]. A recent article demonstrated that older adults with asthma and depression were nearly twice as likely to have poor asthma outcomes across several indicators, including asthma-related ED/urgent care visits, compared to those without depression [11]. The mechanisms responsible for the negative impact of depression on asthma outcomes are not clearly established, and may relate to inflammation, cerebral anatomic changes, autonomic nervous dysfunction, decreased adherence, or ineffective self-management behaviors [12].

Small trials have shown modest benefit of pharmacotherapy and/or behavioral therapy in the treatment of adults with coexisting asthma and depression, though none were exclusively performed in an older population [13–16]. Given the prevalence of depression among older adults, its known effects on asthma, and the potential benefit of therapy, asthma providers should consider screening patients for depression (e.g., with the Geriatric Depression Scale) [17] and treat or refer as appropriate.

Obesity

Like depression, obesity is an asthma comorbidity that may be more problematic in older adults than younger populations. Obese asthma patients have more symptoms, more frequent and severe exacerbations, reduced response to several asthma medications, and decreased quality of life [18]. The mechanisms behind the link between asthma and obesity are beyond the scope of this chapter but include factors such as diet, microbiome shifts, inflammatory and metabolic changes, and genetic factors [18].

Unfortunately, older adults have some of the highest rates of obesity compared to any other age group. Among all age groups, the obesity prevalence in the United States is highest among individuals aged 40–59 years, at approximately 40%. However, those aged 60 and over are a close second at approximately 37% prevalence [19]. Both of these age strata are much higher than individuals aged 20–39 (31%) and those aged 2–19 (17%). As the population of the United States continues to age, this problem has the potential to significantly intensify in the upcoming years.

The clinician caring for an older obese adult with asthma should stress the relationship between the two. For example, obese individuals may have motivation to lose weight, but worry that exercise will provoke or worsen asthma symptoms. The clinician should stress that optimal asthma control will allow the patient to theoretically do more exercise. This, in turn, will promote weight loss and may allow the patient to subsequently achieve an improved level of asthma control with less medication [20, 21].

Menopause and Hormone Replacement Therapy (HRT)

Several studies have documented the effects of hormones such as estrogen and progesterone on airway caliber and asthma exacerbations. A study of 2322 perimenopausal women found the risk of new-onset asthma was 2.4–3.4 times higher compared to premenopausal women [22], and menopause was associated with an accelerated lung function decline [23]. A separate meta-analysis reported that postmenopausal women on HRT had an increased risk of asthma compared to premenopausal women [24]. Conversely, in women with pre-existing asthma, HRT may improve respiratory symptoms and decrease exacerbations [25].

Menopause may also increase the number of asthma exacerbations [26, 27]. There is a spike in exacerbations among women with asthma that occurs at age 50 [28], the mean age of menopause in the United States. This may indicate that sex hormones have a protective effect in asthma, or that fluctuations in hormonal levels can be particularly detrimental. Asthma in women that begins after menopause is frequently severe, nonatopic, and often requires oral corticosteroids for control [29, 30]. The risks and benefits of HRT must be considered, and the asthma-care provider is in a unique position to offer specific information to assist in making decisions about HRT.

Caregiver Roles and Transportation Difficulties

Older adults are ever more frequently taking on greater care-giving roles – whether that of a spouse with significant medical problems, a child who is living at home, or a grandchild while the parents work. Being in a stressful caregiver position has been associated with poorer self-reported health, more negative health behaviors, and greater use of healthcare [31]. It may be beneficial to inquire and acknowledge the challenges that providing care to others entails, and to highlight that to be optimally effective in such a role requires management of one's own health – including asthma.

Transportation can also be problematic for many older adults. Loss of driving privileges can make follow-up care difficult. The asthma provider can help work with senior service agencies, case managers, or social workers to document the need for follow-up care, and may also try to schedule visits on the same day as other medical appointments [32].

Complementary and Alternative Medicine

The use of complementary and alternative medicine (CAM) to manage asthma symptoms occurs in 20–30% of the asthmatic population [33]. An analysis of over 7000 adults above the age of 55 from the Asthma Call Back Survey found that this number was even higher at 39% [34]. The most frequent modalities included breathing exercises, vitamins, and herbal therapy. Other research has shown that older adults with asthma rarely, if ever, discuss CAM with their physician [5]. Therefore, the provider caring for the older adult with asthma should inquire about CAM usage, discuss potential risks/benefits of such therapies as compared to traditional medicine, and discuss how CAM can be used in conjunction with traditional therapies.

Decreased Perception of Breathlessness

An important mechanism to prevent the progression of an asthma exacerbation is early intervention and treatment [35]. Unfortunately, older adults have a decreased perception of airflow obstruction [36, 37]. Altered perception of airflow limitation has also been demonstrated in women as compared to men, although the mechanisms that explain these differences are unclear and may be multifactorial [38, 39]. A study of older individuals found that those with a decreased perception of airflow obstruction had greater medication costs, hospitalizations, and mortality compared to elderly individuals with a better perception of dyspnea [40].

One tool that may help to overcome the decreased perception of breathlessness in older adults is self-monitoring with a peak flow meter (PFM). The current National Institute of Health (NIH) asthma guidelines recommend self-monitoring as an important component of asthma self-management and considers this an "Evidence Level A" recommendation [35]. The guidelines go on to state that "a PFM should be considered for certain subgroups of asthma patients, including those who have a 'poor perception of airflow obstruction'", and that "older patients are more likely to have poor perception of airflow obstruction." Advocating for a PFM to older patients who have an impaired ability to detecting worsening asthma symptoms may be beneficial. However, one study of providing a PFM to all patients with moderate-to-severe asthma above the age of 50 (regardless of their ability to perceive breathlessness) did not improve outcomes [41].

Financial Concerns

The current rate of poverty among adults over the age of 65 is approximately 10%, and this number is expected to rise in the upcoming years [42]. Poverty has numerous detrimental effects on health, such as the inability to afford insurance copays, increased exposure to pollution and/or environmental triggers, and increased psychological stress which worsens asthma. Patients living in poverty often feel ashamed, and few bring up the inability to pay with their provider [43]. Tangible steps that providers can use include: empathetic questions on the ability to afford medications while on a fixed income, prescribing medications with the lowest copay, provision of a list of financial resources, and referral to social work [44].

Conclusion

There are multiple barriers to effective care for older adults with asthma that contribute to the significant morbidity and mortality seen in this age group. Examples include comorbidities, depression, obesity, menopause, caregiver roles,

Table 5.1 Barriers to effective treatment of asthma in older adults

Item	Possible solution
Comorbidities are common among older adults, and can negatively impact asthma	Identify, acknowledge, and address comorbidities where appropriate
Depression is especially problematic to asthma management for older adults	Consider screening, treatment, and/or referral for depression
Obesity is very common, can be more problematic in older adults for asthma	Stress the relationship between obesity and asthma. Discuss how weight loss improves asthma control, which then makes it easier to do additional exercise. Consider dietician referral
Menopause is often associated with asthma exacerbations	The risks and benefits of hormone replacement therapy should be carefully considered in difficult-to-control asthma
Older adults frequently have caregiver roles for their spouse, children, or grandchildren	Acknowledge the challenges, and stress that to be optimally effective, you must take care of your own health
Transportation can be problematic	Work with senior service agencies and social workers; schedule multiple appointments on the same day
Frequent use of complementary and alternative medicine (CAM) for asthma	Discuss risks and benefits of such therapies with your patient; consider how breathing exercises and asthma education can be incorporated
Decreased perception of breathlessness	Inquire if any difficulty in detecting early asthma symptoms; if present, provide a peak flow meter
Financial obstacles to optimal care	Discuss ability to afford meds; prescribe meds with lowest copay; referral to social work when appropriate

transportation, complementary/alternative medicine, perceptions of breathlessness, and financial obstacles. However, many of these can be successfully addressed and remedied by an empathetic clinician who takes time to specifically inquire and work to find solutions (Table 5.1). In this way, caring for the whole patient is possible.

References

1. Su X, Ren Y, Li M, Zhao X, Kong L, Kang J. Prevalence of comorbidities in asthma and non-asthma patients: a meta-analysis. Medicine (Baltimore). 2016;95(22):e3459.
2. Patel MR, Janevic MR, Heeringa SG, Baptist AP, Clark NM. An examination of adverse asthma outcomes in U.S. adults with multiple morbidities. Ann Am Thorac Soc. 2013;10(5): 426–31.
3. Hsu J, Chen J, Mirabelli MC. Asthma morbidity, comorbidities, and modifiable factors among older adults. J Allergy Clin Immunol Pract. 2018;6(1):236–43.
4. Bayliss EA, Steiner JF, Fernald DH, Crane LA, Main DS. Descriptions of barriers to self-care by persons with comorbid chronic diseases. Ann Fam Med. 2003;1(1):15–21.
5. Baptist AP, Deol BB, Reddy RC, Nelson B, Clark NM. Age-specific factors influencing asthma management by older adults. Qual Health Res. 2010;20(1):117–24.
6. Tay TR, Lee J, Radhakrishna N, Hore-Lacy F, Stirling R, Hoy R, et al. A structured approach to specialist-referred difficult asthma patients improves control of comorbidities and enhances asthma outcomes. J Allergy Clin Immunol Pract. 2017;5(4):956–964 e953.

7. Oka A, Hirano T, Yamaji Y, Ito K, Oishi K, Edakuni N, et al. Determinants of incomplete asthma control in patients with allergic rhinitis and asthma. J Allergy Clin Immunol Pract. 2017;5(1):160–4.

8. Asero R. Efficacy of injection immunotherapy with ragweed and birch pollen in elderly patients. Int Arch Allergy Immunol. 2004;135(4):332–5.

9. Epstein TG, Liss GM, Murphy-Berendts K, Bernstein DI. Risk factors for fatal and nonfatal reactions to subcutaneous immunotherapy: national surveillance study on allergen immunotherapy (2008–2013). Ann Allergy Asthma Immunol. 2016;116(4):354–359 e352.

10. Volkert J, Schulz H, Harter M, Wlodarczyk O, Andreas S. The prevalence of mental disorders in older people in Western countries – a meta-analysis. Ageing Res Rev. 2013;12(1):339–53.

11. Patel PO, Patel MR, Baptist AP. Depression and asthma outcomes in older adults: results from the National Health and Nutrition Examination Survey. J Allergy Clin Immunol Pract. 2017;5(6):1691–1697.e1.

12. Wang L, Wang T, Liu S, Liang Z, Meng Y, Xiong X, et al. Cerebral anatomical changes in female asthma patients with and without depression compared to healthy controls and patients with depression. J Asthma. 2014;51(9):927–33.

13. Brown ES, Vornik LA, Khan DA, Rush AJ. Bupropion in the treatment of outpatients with asthma and major depressive disorder. Int J Psychiatry Med. 2007;37(1):23–8.

14. Mancuso CA, Sayles W, Allegrante JP. Randomized trial of self-management education in asthmatic patients and effects of depressive symptoms. Ann Allergy Asthma Immunol. 2010;105(1):12–9.

15. Brown ES, Howard C, Khan DA, Carmody TJ. Escitalopram for severe asthma and major depressive disorder: a randomized, double-blind, placebo-controlled proof-of-concept study. Psychosomatics. 2012;53(1):75–80.

16. Yorke J, Adair P, Doyle AM, Dubrow-Marshall L, Fleming S, Holmes L, et al. A randomised controlled feasibility trial of Group Cognitive Behavioural Therapy for people with severe asthma. J Asthma. 2017;54(5):543–54.

17. Yesavage JA, Brink TL, Rose TL, Lum O, Huang V, Adey M, et al. Development and validation of a geriatric depression screening scale: a preliminary report. J Psychiatr Res. 1982;17(1):37–49.

18. Peters U, Dixon AE, Forno E. Obesity and asthma. J Allergy Clin Immunol. 2018;141(4):1169–79.

19. Arroyo-Johnson C, Mincey KD, Ackermann N, Milam L, Goodman MS, Colditz GA. Racial and ethnic heterogeneity in self-reported diabetes prevalence trends across hispanic subgroups, National Health Interview Survey, 1997–2012. Prev Chronic Dis. 2016;13:E10.

20. Scott HA, Gibson PG, Garg ML, Pretto JJ, Morgan PJ, Callister R, et al. Dietary restriction and exercise improve airway inflammation and clinical outcomes in overweight and obese asthma: a randomized trial. Clin Exp Allergy. 2013;43(1):36–49.

21. Freitas PD, Ferreira PG, Silva AG, Stelmach R, Carvalho-Pinto RM, Fernandes FL, et al. The role of exercise in a weight-loss program on clinical control in obese adults with asthma. A randomized controlled trial. Am J Respir Crit Care Med. 2017;195(1):32–42.

22. Triebner K, Johannessen A, Puggini L, Benediktsdottir B, Bertelsen RJ, Bifulco E, et al. Menopause as a predictor of new-onset asthma: a longitudinal Northern European population study. J Allergy Clin Immunol. 2016;137(1):50–57 e56.

23. Triebner K, Matulonga B, Johannessen A, Suske S, Benediktsdottir B, Demoly P, et al. Menopause is associated with accelerated lung function decline. Am J Respir Crit Care Med. 2017;195(8):1058–65.

24. Zemp E, Schikowski T, Dratva J, Schindler C, Probst-Hensch N. Asthma and the menopause: a systematic review and meta-analysis. Maturitas. 2012;73(3):212–7.

25. Kos-Kudla B, Ostrowska Z, Marek B, Ciesielska-Kopacz N, Kajdaniuk D, Kudla M. Effects of hormone replacement therapy on endocrine and spirometric parameters in asthmatic postmenopausal women. Gynecol Endocrinol. 2001;15(4):304–11.

26. Balzano G, Fuschillo S, Melillo G, Bonini S. Asthma and sex hormones. Allergy. 2001;56(1):13–20.

27. Townsend EA, Miller VM, Prakash YS. Sex differences and sex steroids in lung health and disease. Endocr Rev. 2012;33(1):1–47.
28. Skobeloff EM, Spivey WH, St Clair SS, Schoffstall JM. The influence of age and sex on asthma admissions. JAMA. 1992;268(24):3437–40.
29. Balzano G, Fuschillo S, De Angelis E, Gaudiosi C, Mancini A, Caputi M. Persistent airway inflammation and high exacerbation rate in asthma that starts at menopause. Monaldi Arch Chest Dis. 2007;67(3):135–41.
30. Moore WC, Meyers DA, Wenzel SE, Teague WG, Li H, Li X, et al. Identification of asthma phenotypes using cluster analysis in the Severe Asthma Research Program. Am J Respir Crit Care Med. 2010;181(4):315–23.
31. Son J, Erno A, Shea DG, Femia EE, Zarit SH, Stephens MA. The caregiver stress process and health outcomes. J Aging Health. 2007;19(6):871–87.
32. Dugdale DC, Epstein R, Pantilat SZ. Time and the patient-physician relationship. J Gen Intern Med. 1999;14(Suppl 1):S34–40.
33. Slader CA, Reddel HK, Jenkins CR, Armour CL, Bosnic-Anticevich SZ. Complementary and alternative medicine use in asthma: who is using what? Respirology. 2006;11(4):373–87.
34. Ward CE, Baptist AP. Characteristics of Complementary and Alternative Medicine (CAM) use among older adults with asthma. J Asthma. 2016;53(5):546–52.
35. Joseph CL, Peterson E, Havstad S, Johnson CC, Hoerauf S, Stringer S, et al. A web-based, tailored asthma management program for urban African-American high school students. Am J Respir Crit Care Med. 2007;175(9):888–95.
36. Parameswaran K, Hildreth AJ, Chadha D, Keaney NP, Taylor IK, Bansal SK. Asthma in the elderly: underperceived, underdiagnosed and undertreated; a community survey. Respir Med. 1998;92(3):573–7.
37. Connolly MJ, Crowley JJ, Charan NB, Nielson CP, Vestal RE. Reduced subjective awareness of bronchoconstriction provoked by methacholine in elderly asthmatic and normal subjects as measured on a simple awareness scale. Thorax. 1992;47(6):410–3.
38. Wijnhoven HA, Kriegsman DM, Snoek FJ, Hesselink AE, de Haan M. Gender differences in health-related quality of life among asthma patients. J Asthma. 2003;40(2):189–99.
39. Osborne ML, Vollmer WM, Linton KL, Buist AS. Characteristics of patients with asthma within a large HMO: a comparison by age and gender. Am J Respir Crit Care Med. 1998;157(1):123–8.
40. Ebihara S, Niu K, Ebihara T, Kuriyama S, Hozawa A, Ohmori-Matsuda K, et al. Impact of blunted perception of dyspnea on medical care use and expenditure, and mortality in elderly people. Front Physiol. 2012;3:238.
41. Buist AS, Vollmer WM, Wilson SR, Frazier EA, Hayward AD. A randomized clinical trial of peak flow versus symptom monitoring in older adults with asthma. Am J Respir Crit Care Med. 2006;174(10):1077–87.
42. National Council on Aging. Economic security for seniors facts. https://www.ncoa.org/news/resources-for-reporters/get-the-facts/economic-security-facts/. Accessed 18 Jan 2017.
43. Alexander GC, Casalino LP, Meltzer DO. Patient-physician communication about out-of-pocket costs. JAMA. 2003;290(7):953–8.
44. Hardee JT, Platt FW, Kasper IK. Discussing health care costs with patients: an opportunity for empathic communication. J Gen Intern Med. 2005;20(7):666–9.

Medication Efficacy and Side Effects in Older Asthmatics

6

Pinkus Goldberg

Introduction

As patients age, we often believe that they leave commonly perceived childhood illnesses behind. Asthma has often been thought of as one of these illnesses. In reality, based on national surveillance data in the USA, adults ≥65 years old have had the largest increase in asthma prevalence, with an increase from 6.0% to 8.1% from 2001 to 2010 [1]. Higher rates of hospitalizations, deaths, and mortality are found in older asthmatics compared to younger age groups [1]. As with other age groups, identifying specific triggers and the underlying etiology of the disease, including specific inflammatory mechanisms, is important as it will provide information regarding effective treatment strategies [2–4]. Personalized therapy that takes into account gender, ethnicity, race, occupation, stress levels, obesity, depression, atopic factors, and patient preference should be included in the evaluation and treatment of the older adult asthmatic [4, 5].

Randomized control studies often exclude older adult patients due to their multiple comorbid conditions. Battaglia et al. noted that out of 1909 study subjects, 43.2% were excluded due to a variety of comorbid diseases [2]. Smoking (34.3%), other lung conditions (5.0%), depression/anxiety (3.3%), arrhythmias (2.3%), and coronary artery disease (1.2%) were the most common reasons for exclusion. Patients older than 85 were excluded at an alarming rate of 57.1%. This is important for clinicians to take into account when making asthma treatment decisions based on randomized control studies, as their findings may not be applicable to the older adult population [2, 4]. Polypharmacy in older adults increases drug interaction risk and side effect potential. Memory loss, other

P. Goldberg (✉)
Indiana University School of Medicine, Indianapolis, IN, USA

Internal Medicine, Community Hospitals Health Care System of Indiana, Indianapolis, IN, USA

Allergy Partners of Central Indiana, Indianapolis, IN, USA

© Springer Nature Switzerland AG 2019
T. E. G. Epstein, S. M. Nyenhuis (eds.), *Treatment of Asthma in Older Adults*,
https://doi.org/10.1007/978-3-030-20554-6_6

53

cognitive dysfunctions, metabolic factors, renal insufficiency, and hepatic and musculoskeletal changes of aging will affect the efficacy and safety of therapeutic measures [6, 7].

Efficacy and Side Effects of Asthma Therapies

Oral Corticosteroids

These agents are potentially the most efficacious but also have the highest side effect potential. EPR-3 guidelines mention a trial of oral corticosteroids in some older adults to assess responsiveness to steroids in order to assist with diagnosis. Exacerbations often require daily dosages for a period of time, and a recommended dose is 1 mg/kg of prednisone with a maximum of 50 mg/day [6, 7]. Daily therapy for 7–14 days is usually tolerated if stopped abruptly, but a gradual reduction in dosage or tapering may be needed. Side effects of oral corticosteroids include glucose intolerance, gastrointestinal bleeding (prior disease or surgery), hypertension, mood changes, and depression. These symptoms may be seen with both acute and chronic oral steroid therapy. Common long-term complications include adrenal insufficiency, ocular cataracts, glaucoma, and osteoporosis [6–8]. Lefebvre et al. analyzed data from 3628 long-term corticosteroid users of varying races and ethnicities in a Medicaid population from 6 states in the United States. The average age was 57.6 ± 16.3 years, and they used oral corticosteroids at least ≥5 mg prednisone daily for over 6-month duration (mean duration 3.8 years) [8, 9]. Taking above 6 mg prednisone daily was associated with an increase in complications related to steroid use. Health-related costs were \$2712–\$8560 above those of nonsystemic steroid users [8]. When the data was stratified based on steroid dosing (low: <6 mg/day, medium: >6–12 mg/day, and high: >12 mg/day), a significant incremental increase in side effects was found based on the increasing dose of oral corticosteroids (see Fig. 6.1) [9]. In those over 65 years old, costs were higher by \$518, \$733, and \$1038, respectively, for the low-, medium-, and high-dose systemic steroid groups of patients [8, 10]. Infection and gastrointestinal complications were increased in the medium to higher corticosteroid group. Cardiovascular, gastrointestinal, and infectious risks were also higher in all three steroid groups [8, 9].

Inhaled Corticosteroids

Inhaled corticosteroids (ICS) are the main controller therapy for persistent asthma in the GINA and other guidelines [6, 9–11]. ICS therapy has a broad anti-inflammatory effect, which improves lung function, quality of life, exacerbation risk, symptom control, and mortality related to asthma [8]. Eosinophilic and Type 2 asthma is largely targeted by this therapy and this type of inflammation (atopic) is thought to decrease in older adults [12, 13]. However, two "induced sputum studies" show similar eosinophilia between younger and older patients [13]. The TENOR

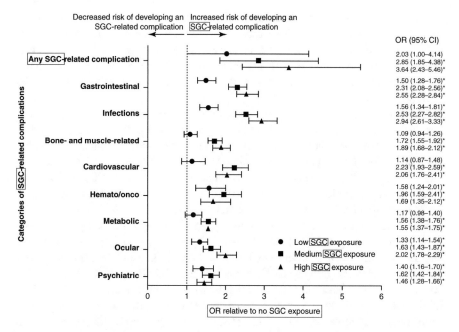

Fig. 6.1 Risk of SGC-related complications by SGC-exposure level relative to no SGC exposure. Error bars represent 95% CIs. *Statistical significance at a level of 0.05. In addition to controlling for key baseline characteristics and time-dependent variables, the GEE model used to estimate the risk of SGC-related complications by SGC exposure controlled for occurrence of the SGC-related complication of interest at baseline. CI confidence interval; GEE generalized estimating equation; OR odds ratio; SGC systemic glucocorticoid. (Reprinted with permission from: Taylor & Francis http://www.informaworld.com Lefebvre et al. [9])

study by Slavin et al. evaluated 566 severe or difficult-to-control asthmatic patients over 65 years of age in a 3-year observational study performed at respiratory specialist sites [14]. These patients had a higher overall usage of inhaled corticosteroids and may have had "more aggressive care" than seen in other older adult studies. Lower healthcare utilization encompassing asthma control, quality of life, and medication usage was noted in the older population versus the younger adults in the study (2912 patients) [15]. Older adults had better control of their asthma ($p < 0.001$) but worse communication with their doctors ($p = 0.02$) [11]. In the observational TENOR study, asthma outcomes such as rehospitalization risk and all-cause mortality were reduced [11, 15]. Despite their effectiveness, ICS therapy is often underutilized in all age groups. Hartert et al. showed that even among patients who were seen on a regular basis prior to a hospital visit, antibiotics and beta agonists were overused, and controller therapies were underused [11, 15].

Although ICS are still a mainstay of treatment in older asthmatics, differences in inflammatory mechanisms for disease may confer differential responses in this age group when compared to younger asthmatics. Eosinophilic and atopic asthma should respond better than neutrophilic inflammatory "TH 17-mediated asthma," the latter of which is increased in the older adult population [10, 11]. Dunn et al.

noted an increase in asthma treatment failures related to age when they retrospectively reviewed ten major asthma trials in an older adult population with mild to moderate asthma [10, 16]. Baptist et al. reviewed these findings and noted that ICS therapy was overpowered statistically versus other controller therapies and therefore non-ICS treatments could not be assessed equally well for efficacy in the older adult population [10, 11].

There are several important considerations when selecting a particular ICS therapy for older patients. ICS treatments with very small-particle-inhaled steroids may be superior to other ICS therapies in the older adult population, who are thought to have more small airways disease. More studies are needed to confirm this hypothesis [10]. Older adults have been noted to suffer a significant deterioration in inhaler technique performance with increasing age when assessed objectively by medical professionals (nurses and pharmacists). On self-assessment, the patients were unaware of their declining inhaler skills, and this was most notable in the over 65 age group [17]. Another study by Melani et al. noted that repeated instruction is needed to maintain correct techniques [18]. It took less time to master dry powder inhalers (DPI) usage than metered dose inhalers (MDI) [18]. Another comparison study between a twice-daily ICS/LABA DPI and a once-daily ICS/LABA DPI product showed a preference for the once-daily product, though both were equally effective [19, 20]. Hirose et al. found a significant difference between male and female patients in inhaler technique in his mid-70s Japanese population [17]. Older adult women had more difficulty "holding their breaths" compared to men [21]. Lower socioeconomic status and cognitive impairment also impacts inhaler technique, and these patients benefit from repeated education on device techniques [20, 22]. Older adults may have difficulty with the use of inhalers due to impaired vision, musculoskeletal disorders, and decreased cognitive function [20, 22]. Park et al. used regression analysis and correlated future asthma exacerbations with low adherence and poor inhalation techniques. Assistance by caregivers over an 8-week course of training improved FEV1 and peak flow measurements in this group of older adults [23]. Nebulized ICS may also be a promising delivery route for these medications in older patients who have difficulty with inhaler techniques [21, 23, 24].

Side effects from ICS therapy may be more pronounced in older adults. Age-related comorbidities and metabolic changes can affect systemic bioavailability [6]. Suppression of the hypothalamic–pituitary axis is a concern, and older patients should receive the lowest-dose ICS with the least bioavailability needed to control their illness. Patients should have a reduction in dosage if well controlled after a 3-month interval [11]. Exhaled nitric oxide or FeNo can be of value in monitoring the response to anti-inflammatory therapy with ICS in older adults [4, 5]. When treating patients with high dosages of ICS, especially women, bone density measurements should be closely followed due to increased fracture risk from osteoporosis. The use of calcium and vitamin D supplementation should be encouraged in these patients. Exercise and avoiding excessive alcohol intake to decrease bone resorption is helpful [11]. Suissa et al. evaluated data from 388,584 patients with respiratory illness over 5 years; data were adjusted for age, comorbidity, gender, and disease severity. The use of ICS was associated with "modest" diabetes progression (rate ratio RR 1.34:95% CI,1.17–1.53) and an increase in the onset of diabetes([RR] 1.34;95% [CI],1.29–1.39) [6, 25]. Antidiabetic medication usage increased in a dose-dependent manner [25]. The greatest risk was in patients using the equivalent of 1000 mcg or more of fluticasone daily. Small but significant risks for developing glaucoma and ocular cataracts have been reported; further studies are recommended [11, 22, 24–28]. Candidiasis in the mouth, throat, and even esophagus has been reported. These conditions as well as dysphonia and hoarseness can worsen if inhaler techniques are not properly implemented, which is more common in older adults [6, 9, 29]. Despite these limitations, ICS are still the preferred controller agents to treat persistent asthma in older adults [11, 29].

Inhaled Bronchodilators

Adrenergic agents starting with inhaled adrenaline have been studied since 1935 as bronchodilators [11]. More selective medicines are now used for a short-acting effect and as long-acting controllers. Short-acting bronchodilators (SABA) are indicated as rescue medications for all types of asthmatic bronchoconstriction, but not for daily use. They have been used extensively in the older adult population with well-established efficacy [6]. The side effect profile for the isomer levalbuterol compared to albuterol is similar in adults, but no specific data are available in older adult patients. These symptoms may include tachycardia, tremor, hyperglycemia, and headache [11]. Nebulized beta 2 agonist bronchodilators may cause dysrhythmias, and the effect is often dose-dependent [6]. Hypokalemia as well as a prolonged QT interval is more often noted in patients with nutritional issues, on insulin, and or diuretics [6]. Despite the previously noted risks, a retrospective one-year study in Japan revealed no increase in pulse rate or hypokalemia when budesonide/formoterol 320/9 mg was used twice daily [9, 29]. Older adults, especially those with concomitant cardiovascular instability, appear more disposed to side effects from beta 2 agonists [11, 28, 30, 31]. Beta 2 receptor responsiveness, density, and affinity may be decreased in older patients [11, 29, 30, 32, 33].

When used as long-acting bronchodilators (LABA), they should be prescribed as an add-on therapy to ICS. The ICS/LABA combination is more effective than the ICS/LTRA (leukotriene receptor antagonist) combination or the doubling of the ICS product dosage [11, 34, 35]. An observational retrospective study obtained via data from Medicare health claims revealed that a salmeterol/fluticasone ICS/LABA combination reduced emergency room and subsequent hospitalization rates by 22% in comparison to those receiving ICS alone [11, 36]. A synergism between ICS and LABAs may take place where the inhaled steroid protects against the "down regulation of the Beta-2 receptors" in response to prolonged usage of the LABA [11]. Monotherapy with LABAs is not recommended due to a higher rate of asthma deaths, but the addition of an ICS at the beginning of therapy alleviates that concern. In the general adult population, a Cochrane meta-analysis found no difference in serious nonfatal or fatal events between the ICS groups and the ICS/LABA groups, including those using either formoterol or salmeterol. Meta-analysis data on older adults is not mentioned [11, 37, 38].

Inhaled Anticholinergics

Cholinergic stimulation leads to bronchoconstriction and blocking the muscarinic receptors, especially M3. This has led to the use of long-acting antimuscarinic antagonists (LAMA) for the treatment of persistent asthma. Selective antagonism of the M3 receptor is most effective in blocking cholinergic bronchoconstriction [11]. Short-acting anticholinergics such as ipratropium bromide have been used in asthma but were inferior to SABAs, perhaps due to nonselective blockade of muscarinic receptors [11]. However, ipratropium bromide, a short-acting antimuscarinic antagonist, has been used in asthma and is often used in an emergency setting for acute exacerbations along with a SABA [6]. Hospital admission rates have been reduced using the combination of antimuscarinic agents and SABAs versus albuterol alone in young adults [6, 39]. It has been speculated that anticholinergic therapy may produce a more pronounced bronchodilator effect compared to beta 2 agonist treatments in older adult patients but the study data did not show that adding a LAMA to a LABA decreased asthma exacerbations, quality of life, or rescue medication use [11, 40, 41].

Efficacy data are limited in older adults, but a study by Kerstjens et al. involving 912 patients up to 75 years of age showed that inhaled tiotropium had proven effectiveness. In this study of poorly controlled asthmatics on ICS/LABA therapy, adding tiotropium modestly improved bronchodilation and "significantly increased the time to the first severe exacerbation" [42]. Other investigators have reported congruent findings in adult patients [11]. Tiotropium, when added to an ICS, was superior to doubling the dose of ICS. Tiotropium was equal in effectiveness to salmeterol plus ICS given twice daily in the improvement of AM peak flow readings [11, 43]. In a study of 472 late middle-age patients where asthma was accompanied by COPD and at least a 10-year history of smoking, tiotropium added to patient therapy improved the degree of bronchoconstriction versus placebo. Magnussen et al. showed that FEV1 significantly improved at the 12-week mark [11, 44]. Further studies are needed in the older adult population in patients with the asthma/COPD overlap syndrome (ACOS) to determine the best treatments for this disease variant [10, 11].

In general, LAMAs are well tolerated in older adult patients [6]. However, dysgeusia may occur and dry mouth may contribute to mucosal damage, poor appetite, denture misfits, speech difficulties, and increased risk of malnutrition. Saliva volume and subsequent antimicrobial activity is reduced, which may increase infection risks in the mouth and pharynx [6]. Increased intraocular pressure, blurred vision, dilated pupils, and closed angle glaucoma are risks to be considered when using high doses of anticholinergics [6, 11]. Long-term cardiovascular risks with LAMAs have been minimally evaluated in asthma, but recent COPD trials are reassuring.

The data from 400 COPD patients with a major cardiac illness history from the UPLIFT (Understanding Potential Long-Term Impacts on Function with Tiotropium) study showed no increase in follow-up cardiac events in the tiotropium cohort compared to the placebo group [11, 45]. Gastrointestinal motility can be slowed, and urinary tract outflow can be decreased in male patients [6, 11]. Paradoxical bronchospasm has been reported with a risk of 0.03 [6, 30]. The potential for inhaled LAMA therapy in older asthmatics appears promising, but current usage is primarily as an add-on therapy to ICS/LABA, where intolerance to LABAs is experienced or other ineffective approaches have been tried [6, 11].

Leukotriene Antagonists

Four pharmaceutical antileukotriene agents are available, including a 5-lipoxygenase inhibitor and three leukotriene-1 antagonists. The medical literature is sparse on using zileuton, a 5-LO inhibitor in older adults [6]. Of the three antileukotrienes available, Zafirlukast has been shown to be less effective in older adults versus younger patients in two studies by Korenblat et al. in 2000 and Creticos et al. in 2002 [11, 46, 47]. However, Pranlukast was studied in 41 patients with mild asthma in comparison to inhaled corticosteroids for an 8-week time frame. Both the inhaled steroid group and the montelukast group showed equivalent improvement from baseline in rescue medication usage, FEV1, and eosinophilic inflammatory measures in the older adult asthmatic group [48]. Studies with montelukast also showed improvement in mild asthma, where adding montelukast to low dosages of budesonide was comparable to doubling the dosage of inhaled steroid. Ye et al. used 800 μg of budesonide in the inhaled steroid group and 400 μg of budesonide with 10 mg of montelukast in the comparison group to show similar efficacy in adults ≥60 years old [11, 49]. Bozek et al. evaluated older adult patients with severe asthma on inhaled steroids versus long-acting beta agonist combinations with or without montelukast over 24 months. Asthma control test scores and days without asthma were significantly higher in the patients on montelukast [50]. A small 17-week double-blind study did not show improvement when montelukast was added to ICS/LABA or LAMA (20%) therapies [51].

LTRAs have theoretical advantages in asthma care for older adults. Advantages of oral therapy include increased adherence compared to inhaled medications, and no dependence on proper inhalation techniques [48]. LFT monitoring will be needed when using zafirlukast and zileuton. Overall, safety and adherence profiles have been acceptable with LTRAs [11, 23, 51].

Theophylline

This pharmaceutical has been used as a bronchodilator since the 1920s. It is a nonselective phosphodiesterase isoenzyme which results in increased levels of cyclic 3′5′guanosine and adenosine monophosphates [6, 11]. Theophylline is a mild bronchodilator compared to beta agonist bronchodilators and has mild anti-inflammatory properties compared to inhaled steroids [11]. These properties may confer some "steroid-sparing" effects in severe asthmatics, and in asthmatics who are steroid resistant [11]. Histone deactylose[2] activity (HDAC[2]) may increase with theophylline usage, which increases steroid sensitivity. This effect is notably seen in smokers even in low therapeutic doses (5 mcg/ml) [6]. Spear et al. evaluated 65 mild to moderate smoking asthmatics where oral theophylline at 400 mg/day in a sustained preparation was added to beclomethasone at 200 mcg/day; this resulted in significant improvements in asthma control and peak flow readings. The mean theophylline serum level in these patients was 4.3 mcg/ml, which is lower than required levels of 10–20 mcg/ml to see a bronchodilator effect [11, 52].

At higher levels of theophylline, the risk of side effects and drug interactions rises, because of its narrow therapeutic window [11]. Pharmacokinetics varies widely among individuals, and theophylline clearance is decreased by 22–35% in the older adult population [6]. Cardiac and hepatic disorders further diminish clearance by 50 percent. Older smokers were noted to have a 50% increase in theophylline clearance, while diet may also affect clearance. High-protein, low-carbohydrate diets, daily consumption of "charcoal-broiled beef," and parenteral nutrition decrease theophylline half-life and increase clearance [6, 52].

Plasma theophylline levels are a safety necessity, but studies have not shown specific problems with aging that prohibit theophylline use in older adults [6]. Drug interactions mediated through the P450 enzyme system or comorbid conditions may affect drug levels [11, 53]. Gastrointestinal symptoms are common and more serious symptoms include palpitations, seizures, arrhythmias, and myocardial infarction (rarely). Using theophylline in a sustained-release low-dose form showed adverse effects in 4.71% of 3810 Japanese patients with a diagnosis of asthma or COPD with an average age of 73.8 years. Most frequent side effects were "nausea (1.05%), loss of appetite (0.56%), hyperuricemia (0.42%), palpitations (0.39%), and elevated alkaline phosphatase levels (0.28%)" [11, 54]. The GINA guidelines place theophylline for use in steps three to five [11]. It can be used in an alternative capacity to inhaled corticosteroids (ICS) in step two or in combination with ICS in step three, although this is rarely done due to the increased potential for side effects. It may be added to medium- or high-dose ICS/LABA combinations in step four or five with close monitoring of plasma levels; it is mostly used as an add-on to ICS/LABA treatment in smoking asthmatics and those with resistance to steroid therapy [6, 7, 11, 52].

Biologic Therapies

Anti-IgE recombinant humanized monoclonal antibody treatment has been used to treat IgE-mediated moderate-to-severe persistent asthma in adults and children with improved asthma outcomes [11]. When an older adult population of veterans who had severe asthma was observed retrospectively, omalizumab increased FEV1 by 280 ml, decreased exacerbations, and improved asthma control based on asthma control test (ACT) scores [11, 55]. Prednisone usage was also markedly decreased in these severe allergic-atopic patients [11, 55]. Although omalizumab is designed to treat atopic asthma, there is some evidence in adults that nonatopic asthma may also respond to this treatment [11, 56]. De Liano et al. obtained data from a multicenter registry analyzing patients from a middle-aged population with atopic (266) and nonatopic (29) severe asthma in Spain [11, 57]. Both groups of patients responded to omalizumab with improvements in asthma exacerbations [11, 58].

In another 41 patients ranging in age from 18- to 70-year-old nonatopic severe asthmatics, omalizumab was shown to decrease "high-affinity IgE receptor (FcERI) expression on basophils and plasmacytoid dendritic cells (pDCs)". In addition, this randomized control study revealed a 250 ml or 9.5% increase in FEV1 [11, 56]. An elevated serum total IgE strongly correlated with staphylococcal enterotoxin-specific IgE (SE-IgE) levels, which are thought to trigger a polyclonal rise in total IgE [11, 58–60]. In addition, crosslinking of FcERI in pDCs is thought to lead to decreased cellular antiviral functioning; omalizumab may therefore have an additional effect in reducing viral asthma exacerbations [11, 61]. The evidence for efficacy of omalizumab in older adult asthmatics is sparse; however, based on available studies, omalizumab appears effective in reducing clinical symptoms and asthma exacerbations, but possibly less than in younger adults [10, 11, 62]. The side effect profile is similar in young adults and in older adults. Hyperglycemia has been reported related to the vials which contain sucrose, and blood sugars may need to be monitored in diabetics [6, 63]. Adverse side effects in older adults are felt to be comparable to those seen in the general population [62].

Anti-interleukin- 5 (IL-5) therapies have been developed to treat severe eosinophilic persistent asthma and include mepolizumab, reslizumab, and benralizumab. Therapy is based on serum eosinophil, not IgE levels [64]. Mepolizumab is approved for the treatment of severe eosinophilic asthma in adults and has been studied in a broad-age range of patients (12–82 years old) [64]. The mepolizumab as adjunctive therapy in patients with severe asthma (MENSA) trial conducted a subanalysis of patients >65 years old and found the rate of asthma exacerbations was decreased by 76% versus placebo [64]. Potential side effects were similar in this cohort of older adults compared to younger adults [64]. Reslizumab also has been shown to reduce asthma exacerbation rates in severe eosinophilic asthma [64, 65]. A post-hoc analysis of two randomized, controlled trials showed that the older adult patients in these reslizumab trials responded with increased FEV1, AQLQ, and ACQ-7 quality-of-life scores compared to the younger adults [65]. Clinical asthma exacerbation frequency also decreased more in the over 65-year-old subgroup compared to the younger patients [65–67]. Further analysis of this data found that those with late-onset (≥40 years old) eosinophilic asthma had greater improvements in lung function and greater decreases in exacerbations than those with early-onset asthma [65]. Side effects were similar for all ages. Benralizumab, in contrast to the anti-IL- 5 antibodies, targets an IL5-alpha-receptor on the eosinophil and has been shown to reduce exacerbations in 18–75-year-old patients with severe persistent eosinophilic asthma. No specific data is as yet available on the older adult subgroup [64].

Other biologic agents under investigation include tralokinumab, lebrikizumab, and dupilumab. Dupilumab blocks IL4 and IL13. It has demonstrated increased lung function and a reduction in severe asthma exacerbations regardless of baseline serum eosinophil levels in a phase 2B study [64, 68]. Dupilumab was approved for the treatment of moderate-to-severe asthma with an eosinophilic phenotype or oral corticosteroid dependent asthma in 2018. The three trials leading to its approval included patients from age 12 and older with a mean age of 48–51 and a SD of 13–15 years [69]. Overall, the asthma biologic therapies have been well tolerated [70]. As they are removed from the body via proteolysis, drug–drug interactions and renal/hepatic impairment are not felt to be significant concerns. These agents target the type 2 immune response and thus may have an effect on parasitic defense systems, which could affect all age groups using these medications [64].

Specific Immunotherapy

Subcutaneous immunotherapy (SCIT) has been available for over 100 years, and several controlled studies have shown it to be efficacious up to 60 years of age. No blinded studies are available in older adults [6]. In their third update, the American Academy of Allergy, Asthma, & Immunology (AAAAI) and American College of Allergy, Asthma, & Immunology (ACAAI) practice parameter recommended that a patient's risk of comorbidities be taken into account when using this therapy [6, 64, 71]. Specific comorbid conditions that may preclude the use of SCIT include unstable or severe angina, significantly decreased lung function, poor asthma control, recent myocardial infarction, uncontrolled hypertension, significant arrhythmia, possibly the use of angiotensin-converting enzyme inhibitors, and beta blockade [6]. Immunotherapy can be started in older adults, and the major consideration is whether they can tolerate epinephrine if needed and survive a systemic reaction [6]. Beta blockers do not increase the risk of reactions to SCIT but make anaphylaxis more difficult to manage [6, 72].

Sublingual Immunotherapy (SLIT) has been evaluated in the older adult population and findings support its efficacy both in retrospective and placebo-controlled studies (the latter in 60 + age group) with specific allergens [73, 74]. SLIT reduces medication use and symptoms while increasing quality of life [73–75]. Sublingual tablets are available for specific immunotherapy with selected grass pollens, ragweed, and house dust mites (HDM) for allergic rhinitis [76]. The safety data when pooled showed the tablets were well tolerated with most adverse reactions being of a mild-to-moderate degree. A greater number of serious adverse events occurred in the not well-controlled asthma group (6%) than in the well-controlled asthma HDM group (2%) [76]. There are no studies specifically evaluating SLIT's effect in the older adult asthmatic population. Various immunotherapy options are available, and their benefits, risks, costs, and management protocols, as well as any patient specific considerations related to safety and adherence, need to be considered before their use in older adults [6, 71, 75].

Other Asthma Therapies

Macrolide antibiotics have been used in treating conditions where neutrophilic inflammation occurs in the airway including bronchiectasis, cystic fibrosis, and diffuse bronchiolitis. Macrolides have anti-inflammatory and immunomodulatory properties in addition to their antibacterial effects. There is evidence that frequent severe asthma exacerbations of a noneosinophilic pathology will respond to chronic maintenance therapy with macrolides, notably azithromycin [77, 78]. Two well-controlled studies showed that selective macrolide therapy was beneficial in non-smokers with severe noneosinophilic asthma [64, 77, 78]. Simpson et al. evaluated nonsmoker asthmatics ranging in age from 27 to 80 (average 60 years) who were given clarithromycin for 8 weeks in a small but well-controlled study. Neutrophils and neutrophil mediators (IL-8) were reduced and quality of life improved [64, 79]. Azithromycin was evaluated in 19–75-year-old patients (mean age 53) with severe noneosinophilic asthma who were nonsmokers or had less than a ten-pack year history of smoking for a 6-month time period. A significant decrease in lower respiratory tract infections and rate of exacerbations was found in this subgroup [66]. Current asthmatic smokers did not respond to the therapy in a study with Azithromycin by Cameron et al. [80] In these studies, the side effect occurrence rate with macrolide add on treatments was equal to the placebo group. Cochrane meta-analysis in 2015 by Kew et al. did not find sufficient data to determine if macrolides are beneficial for severe asthma in general [78].

Bronchial thermoplasty (BT) has been used to treat severe asthma by applying thermal energy via bronchoscopy to decrease swollen bronchial smooth muscle over three procedures, separated by 3–4 weeks [81]. Clinical trials have supported the efficacy of BT in adult patients (Cochrane review – moderate evidence) [82]. Torrega et al. evaluated 429 participants in three studies with a mean age of 39.36 (±11.18) years. Moderate increases in quality of life and decreased asthma exacerbations were reported after 12 months. Respiratory exacerbations during the course of treatment were increased but not after 12 months [82]. Further data are needed to determine the risks and benefits of BT in older adults. See Fig. 6.2.

Complementary/Alternative Medicine

Acupuncture has been used to treat asthma, but scientifically derived data and meta-analysis have not found this treatment modality to be effective [6, 83].

Chiropractic techniques have not been effective in the majority of clinical trials [6, 84, 85]. Breathing control, yoga, hypnosis, and biofeedback have an effect on well-being, but the medical literature has yet to demonstrate a conclusive treatment effect for asthma in general nor in the older asthmatic population [6, 86, 87]. Homeopathy has not shown clinical benefit in prior asthma studies, and no data are available in older adults [6, 88, 89].

Herbal or phytotherapy may be of use in treating asthma, but insufficient evidence is available to make specific recommendations [89]. Lack of consistent

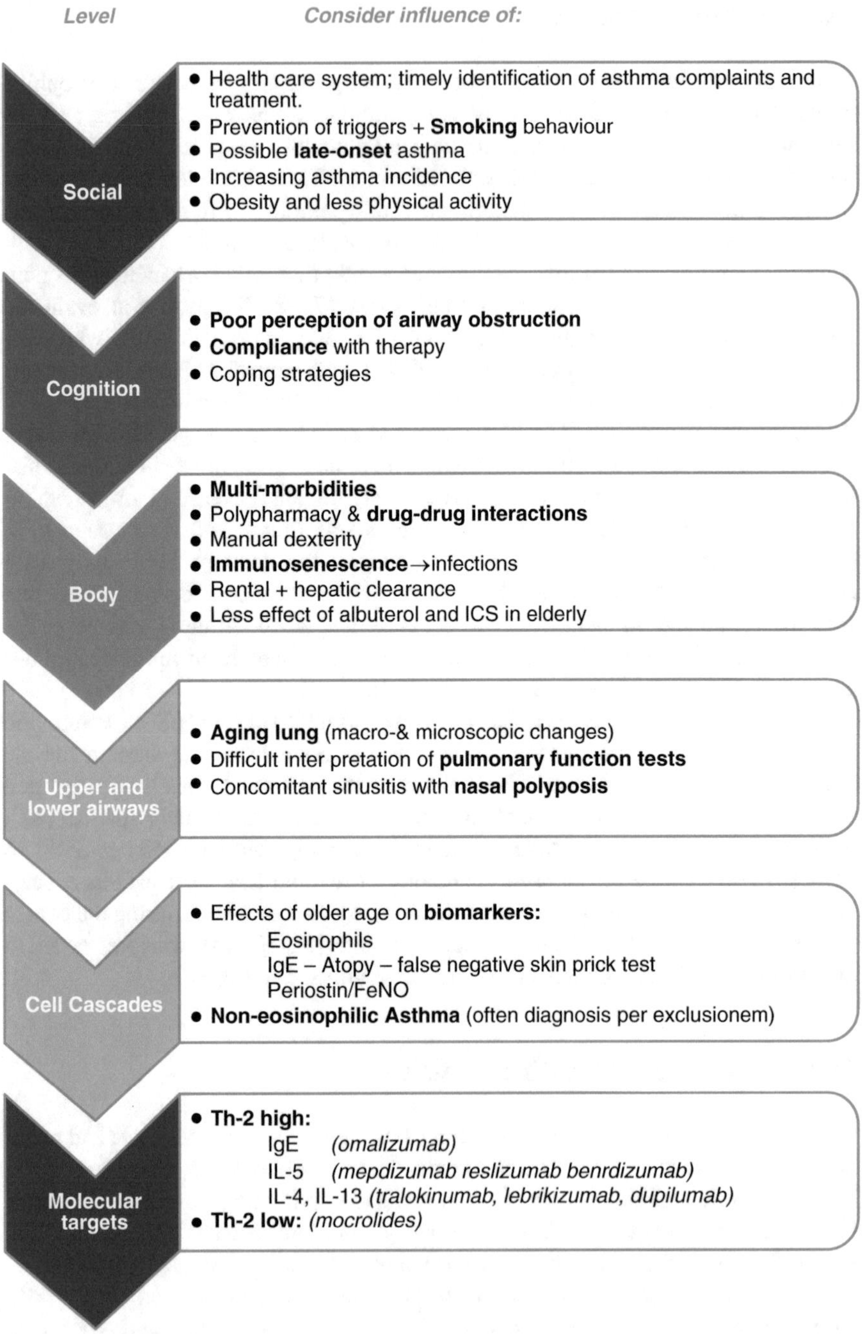

Level   Consider influence of:

Social
- Health care system; timely identification of asthma complaints and treatment.
- Prevention of triggers + **Smoking** behaviour
- Possible **late-onset** asthma
- Increasing asthma incidence
- Obesity and less physical activity

Cognition
- **Poor perception of airway obstruction**
- **Compliance** with therapy
- Coping strategies

Body
- **Multi-morbidities**
- Polypharmacy & **drug-drug interactions**
- Manual dexterity
- **Immunosenescence**→infections
- Rental + hepatic clearance
- Less effect of albuterol and ICS in elderly

Upper and lower airways
- **Aging lung** (macro-& microscopic changes)
- Difficult inter pretation of **pulmonary function tests**
- Concomitant sinusitis with **nasal polyposis**

Cell Cascades
- Effects of older age on **biomarkers:**
    Eosinophils
    IgE – Atopy – false negative skin prick test
    Periostin/FeNO
- **Non-eosinophilic Asthma** (often diagnosis per exclusionem)

Molecular targets
- **Th-2 high:**
    IgE   (omalizumab)
    IL-5   (mepdizumab reslizumab benrdizumab)
    IL-4, IL-13 (tralokinumab, lebrikizumab, dupilumab)
- **Th-2 low:** (mocrolides)

Fig. 6.2 Personalized medicine in elderly asthmatics: defining the target. FeNO nitric oxide in the exhaled breath, ICS inhaled corticosteroids, Ig immunoglobulin, IL interleukin, Th-2 helper cell type 2. (Reprinted with permission from Drugs & Aging: Springer Nature *Targeted Therapy for Older Patients with Uncontrolled Severe Asthma: Current and Future Prospects* by E. W. de Roos, J. C. C. M. in't Veen, G.-J. Braunstahl et al. COPYRIGHT 2016)

production techniques and the lack of studies in the older adult population may lead to undesirable effects, and atopic patients have a greater risk of allergic reactions to these products [6, 90]. Probiotics, prebiotics, and the combination symbiotics are unproven for use in asthma [6, 91].

Conclusion

Healthcare professions are seeing an increasing number of older asthmatic patients. These patients' disease is relatively understudied, and they have more comorbidities and complexity of therapies due to their age. Inhaled steroids, long-acting broncho-dilators, and other therapies need to be employed based on research data for this aging population, although careful monitoring is warranted given less data and increased risk of side effects in older adults for many medications. Adequate evaluation and communication will be the key to effective therapy.

Acknowledgments Rebecca A Goldberg RN, BS Acct., Barbara A. Gushrowski, MLS, Manager of Library Services at Community Health Network, Indianapolis, Indiana.

Potential Conflicts of Interest Consultant and or Speaker for AstraZeneca, Genentech, Boehringer Ingelheim, Circassia, Shire.

References

1. Battaglia S, Benfante A, Scichilone N. Asthma in the older adult: presentation, considerations and clinical management. Expert Rev Clin Immunol. 2015;11(12):1297–308.
2. Battaglia S, et al. Are asthmatics enrolled in randomized trials representative of real-life outpatients? Respiration. 2015;89(5):383–9.
3. Dunn RM, Busse PJ, Wechsler ME. Asthma in the elderly and late-onset adult asthma. Allergy. 2018;73(2):284–94.
4. Bellanti JA, Settipane RA. Atopy, asthma, and the elderly: a paradigm for personalized therapy. Allergy Asthma Proc. 2017;38(3):167–9.
5. Godinho Netto AC, et al. Fraction of exhaled nitric oxide measurements in the diagnoses of asthma in elderly patients. Clin Interv Aging. 2016;11:623–9.
6. Scichilone N, et al. Choosing wisely: practical considerations on treatment efficacy and safety of asthma in the elderly. Clin Mol Allergy. 2015;13(1):7.
7. Horak F, et al. Diagnosis and management of asthma – statement on the 2015 GINA guidelines. Wien Klin Wochenschr. 2016;128(15–16):541–54.
8. Spaggiari L, et al. Exacerbations of severe asthma: a focus on steroid therapy. Acta Biomed. 2014;85(3):205–15.
9. Lefebvre P, et al. Burden of systemic glucocorticoid-related complications in severe asthma. Curr Med Res Opin. 2017;33(1):57–65.
10. Baptist AP, Busse PJ. Asthma over the age of 65: all's well that ends well. J Allergy Clin Immunol Pract. 2018;6(3):764–73.
11. Kim MY, Song WJ, Cho SH. Pharmacotherapy in the management of asthma in the elderly: a review of clinical studies. Asia Pac Allergy. 2016;6(1):3–15.
12. Sin DD, Tu JV. Inhaled corticosteroids and the risk of mortality and readmission in elderly patients with chronic obstructive pulmonary disease. Am J Respir Crit Care Med. 2001;164(4):580–4.
13. Busse PJ, et al. Effect of aging on sputum inflammation and asthma control. J Allergy Clin Immunol. 2017;139(6):1808–1818 e6.

14. Slavin RG, et al. Asthma in older adults: observations from the epidemiology and natural history of asthma: outcomes and treatment regimens (TENOR) study. Ann Allergy Asthma Immunol. 2006;96(3):406–14.
15. Hartert TV, et al. Underutilization of controller and rescue medications among older adults with asthma requiring hospital care. J Am Geriatr Soc. 2000;48(6):651–7.
16. Dunn RM, et al. Impact of age and sex on response to asthma therapy. Am J Respir Crit Care Med. 2015;192(5):551–8.
17. Hira D, et al. Problems of elderly patients on inhalation therapy: difference in problem recognition between patients and medical professionals. Allergol Int. 2016;65(4):444–9.
18. Melani AS, et al. Time required to rectify inhaler errors among experienced subjects with faulty technique. Respir Care. 2017;62(4):409–14.
19. Ishiura Y, et al. A comparison of the efficacy of once-daily fluticasone furoate/vilanterole with twice-daily fluticasone propionate/salmeterol in elderly asthmatics. Drug Res (Stuttg). 2018;68(1):38–44.
20. Turan O, Turan PA, Mirici A. Parameters affecting inhalation therapy adherence in elderly patients with chronic obstructive lung disease and asthma. Geriatr Gerontol Int. 2017;17(6):999–1005.
21. Hirose M, et al. Sex differences in use of inhalants by elderly patients with asthma. Clin Interv Aging. 2015;10:1305–10.
22. Serper M, et al. Health literacy, cognitive ability, and functional health status among older adults. Health Serv Res. 2014;49(4):1249–67.
23. Park HW, et al. Prediction of asthma exacerbations in elderly adults: results of a 1-year prospective study. J Am Geriatr Soc. 2013;61(9):1631–2.
24. Zhou W, Ke H, Li Y. Effect of nebulized corticosteroids on long-term poorly controlled asthma in elderly patients. Chin J Geriatr. 2015;34(7):711–4.
25. Suissa S, Kezouh A, Ernst P. Inhaled corticosteroids and the risks of diabetes onset and progression. Am J Med. 2010;123(11):1001–6.
26. Garbe E, Suissa S, LeLorier J. Association of inhaled corticosteroid use with cataract extraction in elderly patients. JAMA. 1998;280(6):539–43.
27. Ernst P, et al. Low-dose inhaled and nasal corticosteroid use and the risk of cataracts. Eur Respir J. 2006;27(6):1168–74.
28. Leone FT, et al. Systematic review of the evidence regarding potential complications of inhaled corticosteroid use in asthma: collaboration of American College of Chest Physicians, American Academy of Allergy, Asthma, and Immunology, and American College of Allergy, Asthma, and Immunology. Chest. 2003;124(6):2329–40.
29. Kagohashi K, et al. Long-term safety of budesonide/formoterol for the treatment of elderly patients with bronchial asthma. Exp Ther Med. 2014;7(4):1005–9.
30. Gupta P, O'Mahony MS. Potential adverse effects of bronchodilators in the treatment of airways obstruction in older people: recommendations for prescribing. Drugs Aging. 2008;25(5):415–43.
31. Bellia V, et al. Asthma in the elderly: mortality rate and associated risk factors for mortality. Chest. 2007;132(4):1175–82.
32. Connolly MJ. Ageing, late-onset asthma and the beta-adrenoceptor. Pharmacol Ther. 1993;60(3):389–404.
33. Connolly MJ, et al. Impaired bronchodilator response to albuterol in healthy elderly men and women. Chest. 1995;108(2):401–6.
34. Chauhan BF, Ducharme FM. Addition to inhaled corticosteroids of long-acting beta2-agonists versus anti-leukotrienes for chronic asthma. Cochrane Database Syst Rev. 2014;1:CD003137.
35. O'Byrne PM, et al. Increasing doses of inhaled corticosteroids compared to adding long-acting inhaled beta2-agonists in achieving asthma control. Chest. 2008;134(6):1192–9.
36. Stanford RH, et al. Effect of combination fluticasone propionate and salmeterol or inhaled corticosteroids on asthma-related outcomes in a medicare-eligible population. Am J Geriatr Pharmacother. 2012;10(6):343–51.

37. Cates CJ, et al. Regular treatment with formoterol and inhaled steroids for chronic asthma: serious adverse events. Cochrane Database Syst Rev. 2013;6:CD006924.
38. Cates CJ, et al. Regular treatment with salmeterol and inhaled steroids for chronic asthma: serious adverse events. Cochrane Database Syst Rev. 2013;3:CD006922.
39. Rodrigo GJ, Rodrigo C. First-line therapy for adult patients with acute asthma receiving a multiple-dose protocol of ipratropium bromide plus albuterol in the emergency department. Am J Respir Crit Care Med. 2000;161(6):1862–8.
40. Sobieraj DM, et al. Association of inhaled corticosteroids and long-acting muscarinic antagonists with asthma control in patients with uncontrolled, persistent asthma: a systematic review and meta-analysis. JAMA. 2018;319(14):1473–84.
41. Slawson D. Long-acting muscarinic antagonists plus inhaled steroids is equal to long-acting beta-agonists plus inhaled steroids. Am Fam Physician. 2018;98(8).: Online
42. Kerstjens HA, et al. Tiotropium in asthma poorly controlled with standard combination therapy. N Engl J Med. 2012;367(13):1198–207.
43. Peters SP, et al. Tiotropium bromide step-up therapy for adults with uncontrolled asthma. N Engl J Med. 2010;363(18):1715–26.
44. Magnussen H, et al. Improvements with tiotropium in COPD patients with concomitant asthma. Respir Med. 2008;102(1):50–6.
45. Tashkin DP, et al. Cardiac safety of tiotropium in patients with cardiac events: a retrospective analysis of the UPLIFT(R) trial. Respir Res. 2015;16:65.
46. Korenblat PE, et al. Effect of age on response to zafirlukast in patients with asthma in the Accolate Clinical Experience and Pharmacoepidemiology Trial (ACCEPT). Ann Allergy Asthma Immunol. 2000;84(2):217–25.
47. Creticos P, et al. Loss of response to treatment with leukotriene receptor antagonists but not inhaled corticosteroids in patients over 50 years of age. Ann Allergy Asthma Immunol. 2002;88(4):401–9.
48. Trinh HK, et al. Leukotriene receptor antagonists for the treatment of asthma in elderly patients. Drugs Aging. 2016;33(10):699–710.
49. Ye YM, et al. Addition of montelukast to low-dose inhaled corticosteroid leads to fewer exacerbations in older patients than medium-dose inhaled corticosteroid monotherapy. Allergy Asthma Immunol Res. 2015;7(5):440–8.
50. Bozek A, et al. Montelukast as an add-on therapy to inhaled corticosteroids in the treatment of severe asthma in elderly patients. J Asthma. 2012;49(5):530–4.
51. Columbo M. Asthma in the elderly: a double-blind, placebo-controlled study of the effect of montelukast. Asthma Res Pract. 2017;3:3.
52. Spears M, et al. Effect of low-dose theophylline plus beclometasone on lung function in smokers with asthma: a pilot study. Eur Respir J. 2009;33(5):1010–7.
53. Barnes PJ. Theophylline. Am J Respir Crit Care Med. 2013;188(8):901–6.
54. Ohta K, et al. A prospective clinical study of theophylline safety in 3810 elderly with asthma or COPD. Respir Med. 2004;98(10):1016–24.
55. Verma P, Randhawa I, Klaustermeyer WB. Clinical efficacy of omalizumab in an elderly veteran population with severe asthma. Allergy Asthma Proc. 2011;32(5):346–50.
56. Garcia G, et al. A proof-of-concept, randomized, controlled trial of omalizumab in patients with severe, difficult-to-control, nonatopic asthma. Chest. 2013;144(2):411–9.
57. de Llano LP, Vennera Mdel C, Alvarez FJ, Medina JF, Borderdas L, Pellicer C, Gonzalez H, Gullon JA, Martinez-Moragon E, Sabadell C, Zamarro S, Picado C. Effects of omalizumab in non-atopic asthma; results froma a Spanish multicenter registry. J Asthma. 2013;144:411–9.
58. Song WJ, et al. Staphylococcal enterotoxin sensitization in a community-based population: a potential role in adult-onset asthma. Clin Exp Allergy. 2014;44(4):553–62.
59. Song WJ, et al. Staphylococcal enterotoxin IgE sensitization in late-onset severe eosinophilic asthma in the elderly. Clin Exp Allergy. 2016;46(3):411–21.
60. Bachert C, Gevaert P, van Cauwenberge P. Staphylococcus aureus enterotoxins: a key in airway disease? Allergy. 2002;57(6):480–7.

61. Tversky JR, et al. Human blood dendritic cells from allergic subjects have impaired capacity to produce interferon-alpha via Toll-like receptor 9. Clin Exp Allergy. 2008;38(5):781–8.
62. Maykut RJ, Kianifard F, Geba GP. Response of older patients with IgE-mediated asthma to omalizumab: a pooled analysis. J Asthma. 2008;45(3):173–81.
63. Yalcin AD, et al. Omalizumab (anti-IgE) therapy increases blood glucose levels in severe persistent allergic asthma patients with diabetes mellitus: 18 month follow-up. Clin Lab. 2014;60(9):1561–4.
64. de Roos EW, et al. Targeted therapy for older patients with uncontrolled severe asthma: current and future prospects. Drugs Aging. 2016;33(9):619–28.
65. Bernstein DI, Mansfield L, Zangrilli J, Garin M. Efficacy of reslizumab in older patients (> 65 years) with asthma and elevated blood eosinophils: results from a pooled analysis of two phase 3, placebo-controlled trials. J Allergy Clin Immunol. 2016;137(2):AB86.
66. Brusselle GG, et al. Azithromycin for prevention of exacerbations in severe asthma (AZISAST): a multicentre randomised double-blind placebo-controlled trial. Thorax. 2013;68(4):322–9.
67. Brusselle G, et al. Reslizumab in patients with inadequately controlled late-onset asthma and elevated blood eosinohils. Pulm Pharmacol Ther. 2017;43:39–45.
68. Wenzel S, et al. Dupilumab efficacy and safety in adults with uncontrolled persistent asthma despite use of medium-to-high-dose inhaled corticosteroids plus a long-acting beta2 agonist: a randomised double-blind placebo-controlled pivotal phase 2b dose-ranging trial. Lancet. 2016;388(10039):31–44.
69. Dupixent (dupilumb) injection 200 mg. 300mg Full Prescribing, S. Genzyme, editor; 2018.
70. Israel E, Reddel HK. Severe and difficult-to-treat asthma in adults. N Engl J Med. 2017;377(10):965–76.
71. Cox L, Nelson H, Lockey R. Allergen immunotherapy: a practice parameter. J Allergy Clin Immunol. 2011;127(1)(3rd update): 51–55.
72. Lang DM. Do beta-blockers really enhance the risk of anaphylaxis during immunotherapy? Curr Allergy Asthma Rep. 2008;8(1):37–44.
73. Marogna M, et al. Sublingual immunotherapy for allergic respiratory disease in elderly patients: a retrospective study. Eur Ann Allergy Clin Immunol. 2008;40(1):22–9.
74. Bozek A, et al. Grass pollen sublingual immunotherapy: a double-blind, placebo-controlled study in elderly patients with seasonal allergic rhinitis. Am J Rhinol Allergy. 2014;28(5):423–7.
75. Canonica GW, et al. Sublingual immunotherapy: World Allergy Organization position paper 2013 update. World Allergy Organ J. 2014;7(1):6.
76. Emminger W, et al. The SQ house dust mite SLIT-Tablet is well tolerated in patients with house dust mite respiratory allergic disease. Int Arch Allergy Immunol. 2017;174(1):35–44.
77. Albert RK, et al. Azithromycin for prevention of exacerbations of COPD. N Engl J Med. 2011;365(8):689–98.
78. Kew KM, et al. Macrolides for chronic asthma. Cochrane Database Syst Rev. 2015;9:CD002997.
79. Simpson JL, et al. Clarithromycin targets neutrophilic airway inflammation in refractory asthma. Am J Respir Crit Care Med. 2008;177(2):148–55.
80. Cameron EJ, Chaudhuri R, Mair F, McSharry C, Greenlaw N, Weir CJ, et al. Randomized controlled trial of azithomycin in smokers with asthma. Eur Respir J. 2013;42(5):1412–5.
81. Burn J, et al. Procedural and short-term safety of bronchial thermoplasty in clinical practice: evidence from a national registry and Hospital Episode Statistics. J Asthma. 2017;54(8):872–9.
82. Torrego A, et al. Bronchial thermoplasty for moderate or severe persistent asthma in adults. Cochrane Database Syst Rev. 2014;3:CD009910.
83. Wechsler ME, et al. Active albuterol or placebo, sham acupuncture, or no intervention in asthma. N Engl J Med. 2011;365(2):119–26.
84. Nielsen NH, et al. Chronic asthma and chiropractic spinal manipulation: a randomized clinical trial. Clin Exp Allergy. 1995;25(1):80–8.
85. Balon J, et al. A comparison of active and simulated chiropractic manipulation as adjunctive treatment for childhood asthma. N Engl J Med. 1998;339(15):1013–20.

86. Huntley A, White AR, Ernst E. Relaxation therapies for asthma: a systematic review. Thorax. 2002;57(2):127–31.
87. Hackman RM, Stern JS, Gershwin ME. Hypnosis and asthma: a critical review. J Asthma. 2000;37(1):1–15.
88. Reilly D, et al. Is evidence for homoeopathy reproducible? Lancet. 1994;344(8937):1601–6.
89. Lewith GT, et al. Use of ultramolecular potencies of allergen to treat asthmatic people allergic to house dust mite: double blind randomised controlled clinical trial. BMJ. 2002;324(7336):520.
90. Bielory L. Adverse reactions to complementary and alternative medicine: ragweed's cousin, the coneflower (echinacea), is "a problem more than a sneeze". Ann Allergy Asthma Immunol. 2002;88(1):7–9.
91. Vliagoftis H, et al. Probiotics for the treatment of allergic rhinitis and asthma: systematic review of randomized controlled trials. Ann Allergy Asthma Immunol. 2008;101(6):570–9.

Treatment of Asthma in Older Adults with Significant Medical Comorbidities

7

Anil Nanda and Anita N. Wasan

Introduction

Comorbid medical conditions can significantly impact the management of asthma in the older adult [1]. Older adults with asthma have a higher mortality rate than younger individuals [2]. In 2009, approximately 12% of patients with asthma were older adults; however, more than 50% of asthma-related deaths occurred in patients older than 65 years [3]. Asthma hospitalization rates among patients over 65 years were three times higher than younger patients [3]. In one study involving over 14,000 patients aged 65 and older with asthma, increased asthma-related emergency department and urgent care visits were associated with having comorbid medical conditions [4]. Compared with other age groups, asthmatics above the age of 55 had significantly more comorbid conditions, such as hypertension, diabetes, congestive heart failure, depression, and obesity [2]. Having medical comorbidities has also been associated with more difficult-to-control asthma [5]. The true prevalence and impact of comorbid conditions in older adults with asthma is not well understood as they have been excluded in many population-based studies. Given that the population is aging worldwide, there is a vital need for additional studies on the impact of these comorbidities in older adults [2].

A. Nanda (✉)
Asthma and Allergy Center, Lewisville and Flower Mound, TX, USA

Division of Allergy and Immunology, University of Texas Southwestern Medical Center, Dallas, TX, USA

A. N. Wasan
Allergy and Asthma Center, McLean, VA, USA

© Springer Nature Switzerland AG 2019
T. E. G. Epstein, S. M. Nyenhuis (eds.), *Treatment of Asthma in Older Adults*,
https://doi.org/10.1007/978-3-030-20554-6_7

The Impact of Co-morbid Pulmonary Disease on Asthma and Treatment in Older Adults

Asthma COPD overlap syndrome (ACOS), although controversial, is a specific entity that has been described [6]. These patients, a majority of whom are older adults, tend to have lower quality of life, greater symptom burden, and more hospitalizations than those with only COPD or asthma [6]. The pathophysiology of COPD and asthma may impact therapy choices. Despite multiple phenotypes, asthma is thought to be more of an eosinophilic process, and COPD is thought to be more of a neutrophilic process [7].

Although no specific guidelines exist, treatment of ACOS usually involves the initiation of asthma therapy with inhaled corticosteroids, with addition of long-acting β-agonist (LABA) or long-acting muscarinic antagonist (LAMA) in combination or alone [7]. Studies have demonstrated efficacy of inhaled corticosteroid and LABA therapy in COPD patients with peripheral blood eosinophilia [8]. Medical therapies for COPD involve short- and long-acting bronchodilators as well as inhaled corticosteroids [9]. Other treatment options for more advanced disease include oxygen therapy and pulmonary rehabilitation, as well as inhaled corticosteroids [9].

As smoking is a major risk factor for COPD, smoking cessation is a cornerstone of therapy [9]. Studies have shown that older adult asthma patients have a higher incidence of smoking than their younger counterparts [1, 10]. Tobacco cessation should be addressed by healthcare providers, as even brief physician advice has shown to promote tobacco cessation [11]. When addressing smoking cessation, assessing patient severity of tobacco dependence is one of the first steps [11]. Discussing the benefits of smoking cessation is another important step, as the potential for improved survival is underappreciated by many patients [11]. Finally, the addition of pharmacologic therapy is sometimes necessary to achieve smoking cessation. Commonly used medications for smoking cessation include nicotine replacement therapy through transdermal, oral, and inhalation routes [11]; varenicline, a partial agonist of α-4, β-2 nicotinic acetylcholine receptor; and bupropion, a reuptake inhibitor of dopamine and norepinephrine [11]. Older adults may be more susceptible to side effects of these medications, including nausea, sleep issues, and vivid dreaming with varenicline, and seizures with bupropion [11].

The Impact of Comorbid Cardiac Disease on Asthma and Treatment in Older Adults

It has been postulated that there is an association between asthma/ACOS and cardiovascular disease [12]. A population-based cohort study was performed in patients above age 40 years to explore a possible relationship between ACOS and cardiovascular disease (coronary artery disease, cardiac arrhythmia, and heart failure) [12]. ACOS was associated with an overall higher cardiovascular disease risk, even without any prior history of cardiovascular risk factors including diabetes, hypertension, and hyperlipidemia [12]. In addition, patients with comorbid cardiovascular disease, especially congestive heart failure, may mistake their symptoms with asthma and vice versa. Patients should be well educated on the symptoms of each condition as well as overlapping symptoms and taught self-management skills (such as checking peak flows and daily weights) that may help them discern between the two diseases. Two common medications in patients with cardiovascular disease include angiotensin-converting enzyme (ACE) inhibitors and β-blockers. Some studies have shown an increase in anaphylaxis risk in patients on these medications, and a careful review of the risks and benefits should be undertaken in the older asthma patient on these medications, including the initiation of allergen immunotherapy [13]. In one study, patients with ACOS who used selective β1-blockers, such as atenolol, had a higher risk of cardiovascular disease [13]. Beta-agonist therapy in older adults with asthma can be potentially associated with more severe hypokalemia, QT interval prolongation, tachycardia, and tremor [14]. With regard to the potential risk of β-blockers in the treatment of hypertension in asthma patients, the selection of cardioselective beta-blockers may be beneficial [15]. In patients with diabetes, oral steroids may increase serum glucose levels. Given all of the above issues, including issues with β-agonist therapy, biologic therapies for asthma may be a good therapeutic option for patients who cannot tolerate other medications due to comorbid cardiac disease or diabetes [16, 17].

The Impact of Comorbid GERD on Asthma and Treatment in Older Adults

The prevalence of GERD in asthma patients is estimated to be between 42% and 69% [18]. Laryngopharyngeal reflux (LPR) can also occur [19]. Older adults may not experience typical reflux symptoms of heartburn or acidity but may present with anorexia, weight loss, anemia, or dysphagia [19]. Given the potentially atypical symptoms on presentation, older adults with GERD may benefit from a comprehensive gastroesophageal evaluation, including pH-probe and esophagogastroduodenoscopy rather than only empiric proton pump inhibitor therapy [19]. Once the diagnosis is made, behavioral and lifestyle changes can be implemented, including smoking cessation, weight loss, alcohol avoidance, and avoiding late meals [19]. Antacids should be used with caution due to potentially high amounts of sodium and calcium [19]. Histamine 2 receptor (H-2) antagonists similarly should be used with caution as they can lead to mental status changes in patients with liver and renal impairment [19]. Cimetidine, an H-2 receptor antagonist, can also impede liver enzyme metabolism, leading to interactions with common medications among older adults, including warfarin, cyclobenzaprine, and clozapine [19]. The gold standard medication to treat GERD, proton pump inhibitors, has been associated with dementia in older adults; however, further studies are needed [19]. Prokinetic agents such as metoclopramide are generally not recommended in older patients due to potential confusion, drowsiness, and tardive dyskinesia [19]. Laparoscopic surgery may be a viable option to avoid side effects from the above medications as well as in patients in whom medical therapy was ineffective [19].

The Impact of Depression and Dementia on Asthma and Treatment in Older Adults

Quality of life in older adult asthmatics is significantly impacted by depression as well as dementia [1]. The prevalence of depression in older adults has been estimated to be at 20% [6]. One study examined the psychological, demographic, and physiologic characteristics associated with asthma in adults over 65 years, using the Center for Epidemiologic Studies Depression Scale (CES-D8) and Short-Form Health Survey (SF) [20]. Elevated depression scores were found and correlated with reduced quality of life and asthma control scores [20]. In addition, the risk of depression increases with the presence of other medical conditions [20]. One study of 179 older adults with asthma found that patients had higher symptoms of depression and more negative feelings regarding their lives than patients without asthma [21]. Another study involving 1233 older asthma patients in Italy found that depression and state of mood were indicators of asthma mortality [22]. Cognitive impairments and poorer perceptions of dyspnea in older adults may also further complicate adherence [14, 23].

It has been postulated that the stigma associated with depression, cognitive impairments, and mental illness as well as misunderstanding of asthma by caregivers and patients may contribute to the inadequate treatment of depression in older patients [24]. Providers should screen for depression using validated assessment tools [25]. With regard to treatment of depression, cognitive behavioral therapy and pulmonary rehabilitation have been shown to improve both depression symptoms and quality of life in relatively short-term interventions [24]. The value of antidepressant therapy for depression in older patients with COPD and asthma has been overall inconclusive [24]. Collaborative care involving psychiatry specialists in addition to patient-directed education has been shown to decrease depression symptoms in older patients, regardless of medical comorbidities [26]. Decreased cognition can potentially impair the ability of patients to properly self-administer their asthma medications. Improved recognition and treatment of depression and cognitive impairment in older adults are likely to improve asthma-related outcomes. If significant cognitive impairments cannot be medically treated, then other interventions such as home healthcare and institutional care may be evaluated.

The Impact of Rhinitis and Sinusitis on Asthma and Treatment in Older Adults

Rhinitis is an important risk factor for developing asthma and can also be a significant contributing factor to lack of asthma control [27]. Allergic and nonallergic rhinitis affects approximately 32% of older adults [28]. Types of rhinitis in older adults include allergic rhinitis, nonallergic rhinitis, atrophic rhinitis, and drug-induced rhinitis [29]. Triggers of rhinitis include structural changes of the nasal passages, weakening of septal cartilage, and atrophy of the mucosal epithelium [29]. In addition, studies have shown that sinusitis is more common in older asthma patients compared with younger asthma patients [10, 30]. A decrease in mucosal blood flow can also be associated with aging [29]. An increase in cholinergic activity in nostrils with age can also cause an increase in both rhinitis and postnasal drainage [29]. Individualized environmental controls should be initiated in all patients. Cetirizine has shown effectiveness in alleviating upper and lower airway issues in those patients who have both allergic rhinitis and asthma [27]. Optimal rhinitis and chronic sinusitis treatment with a variety of other agents including intranasal corticosteroids and leukotriene antagonists can help decrease asthma exacerbations and beta-agonist use [27]. Allergen immunotherapy is also a viable option, as this may potentially decrease the use of other medications, further alleviating the burden of polypharmacy.

The Impact of Obesity on Asthma and Treatment in Older Adults

There is a link between obesity and asthma, although few studies have examined the role of obesity in older adults with asthma [31, 32]. Obesity rates in older adults are rising at a greater rate than most age groups [33]. In one study involving 675 older individuals with asthma, obesity was a significant predictor of increased overall healthcare cost [34]. Another study involving 437 older adults with asthma found no significant association between obesity and lower Asthma Control Questionnaire (ACQ) or Mini Asthma Quality of Life Questionnaire (Mini-AQLQ) scores [32]. Conversely, being underweight in older age may also have negative ramifications; this was seen in a study of 1233 older asthmatic patients in Italy, where having a body mass index (BMI) less than 22 kg/m [2] was associated with increased mortality [22]. Obese patients may not respond as well to asthma controller medications, as they may have differing cellular reactions to corticosteroids, due to altered signaling proteins, including MKP1 [35]. In those older asthma patients who are obese, therapies for weight loss, such as exercise, diet change, and treatment of potential sleep apnea should be initiated [35]. Exercise has also been shown to improve quality of life in older asthma patients [36].

The Impact of Polypharmacy on Asthma and Treatment in Older Adults

Polypharmacy, a major risk-factor in older asthma patients, impacts overall healthcare in this population [37]. Many studies have defined polypharmacy as five or more medications; older patients having two chronic medical conditions will usually surpass this threshold [38]. Approximately 47% of older patients using at least one prescription medication used over the counter medications as well, and 54% used a dietary supplement [38]. Many older adults with asthma use complementary and alternative medications, and they rarely talk with their health-care provider regarding their use [6].

Drug–drug interactions are a common cause of adverse drug reactions [38]. As many as 35% and 40% of older outpatients and inpatients, respectively, experience an adverse drug reaction [38]. Well-designed multidisciplinary approaches to reduce polypharmacy in older patients have revealed an improvement in overall quality of prescribing practices [38]. A detailed review of all medications, including prescription, over the counter, and all complementary and alternative preparations, should be undertaken at each office visit.

The Impact of Musculoskeletal Comorbidities on Asthma in Older Adults

Many older patients have multiple musculoskeletal conditions, including osteoarthritis, and this can impact the use of asthma inhalers [39, 40]. The Asthma Beliefs and Literacy in the Elderly (ABLE) study involved participation of older adults (>60 years of age) with asthma in the investigation of treatment adherence, including inhalers [39]. MDI inhalers require an increased level of physical coordination and dexterity as compared to DPI inhalers, and it is postulated that older patients with asthma may thus have more challenges with MDI medications [39]. To combat these issues with inhalers, a teach-to-goal technique may be used, instructing patients on self-care skills and demonstrating proper medication technique [39]. Spacers may also be used to aid in MDI use [41].

The Impact of Other Comorbid Medical Conditions on Asthma in Older Adults

There are multiple other comorbidities that can affect older patients with asthma. Having an enlarged prostate or glaucoma can impact the potential for side effects with anticholinergic therapies, including therapies for asthma. Two studies evaluated the effect of anticholinergic medications on functional status in older patients [42]. One study, evaluating 544 older men from a Connecticut Veterans Longitudinal Cohort, revealed that cumulative anticholinergic exposure was associated with poorer functional status [42]. An analysis of 304 patients in a palliative care trial also revealed a lower functional status in patients on anticholinergic medications [42]. Menopause has also been shown to be associated with an increased risk of asthma exacerbations [6].

Conclusion

In summary, older adults with asthma tend to have more severe disease, with comorbid conditions further exacerbating the asthma [43]. Additional measures may be utilized in the treatment of asthma in older adults with multiple comorbidities including the use of validated questionnaires to increase the detection of comorbidities associated with asthma [44]. Awareness and treatment of these multiple medical comorbidities are essential to improving asthma care in the older adult population.

References

1. Hanania N, King M, Braman S, Saltoun C, Wise R, Enright P, et al. Asthma in the elderly: current understanding and future research needs-a report of a National Institute on Aging (NIA) workshop. J Allergy Clin Immunol. 2011;128:s4–24.
2. Tsai C, Lee W, Hanania N, Camargo C. Age-related differences in clinical outcomes for acute asthma in the United States, 2006–2008. J Allergy Clin Immunol. 2012;129:1252–8.
3. Soones T, Lin J, Wolf M, O'Conor R, Martynenko M, Wisnivesky J, et al. Pathways linking health literacy, health beliefs, and cognition to medication adherence in older adults with asthma. J Allergy Clin Immunol. 2017;139:804–9.
4. Hsu J, Chen J, Mirabelli M. Risk factors associated with asthma-related emergency department and urgent care visits among older adults. J Allergy Clin Immunol. 2017;139:AB202.
5. Hekking P, Amelink M, Wener R, Bouvy M, Bel E. Comorbidities in difficult-to-control asthma. J Allergy Clin Immunol Pract. 2017;17:473–7.
6. Baptist A, Busse P. Asthma over the age of 65: all's well that ends well. J Allergy Clin Immunol Pract. 2018;6:764–73.
7. Desai M, Oppenheimer J, Tashkin D. Asthma-chronic obstructive pulmonary disease overlap syndrome: what we know and what we need to find out. Ann Allergy Asthma Immunol. 2017;118:241–5.
8. Siddiqui S, Guasconi A, Vestbo J, et al. Blood eosinophils: a biomarker of response to extrafine beclomethasone/formoterol in chronic obstructive pulmonary disease. Am J Respir Crit Care Med. 2015;192:523–5.
9. Gooneratne N, Patel N, Corcoran A. Chronic obstructive pulmonary disease diagnosis and management in older adults. J Am Geriatr Soc. 2010;58:1153–62.
10. Diette G, Krishnan J, Dominici F, Haponik E, Skinner E, Steinwachs D, et al. Asthma in older patients: factors associated with hospitalization. Arch Intern Med. 2002;162:1123–32.
11. Baldassarri S, Toll B, Leone F. A comprehensive approach to tobacco dependence interventions. J Allergy Clin Immunol. 2015;3:481–8.
12. Yeh J, Wei Y, Lin C, Hsu W. Association of asthma-chronic obstructive pulmonary disease overlap syndrome with coronary artery disease, cardiac dysrhythmia and heart failure: a population-based retrospective cohort study. BMJ Open. 2017;7:1–9.
13. Coop C, Schapira R, Freeman T. Are ACE inhibitors and beta-blockers dangerous in patients at risk for anaphylaxis? J Allergy Clin Immunol Pract. 2017;5:1207–11.
14. Battaglia S, Benfante A, Spatafora M, Scichilone N. Asthma in the elderly: a different disease? Breathe. 2016;12:18–28.
15. Dart R, Gollub S, Lazar J, Nair C, Schroeder D, Woolf S. Treatment of systemic hypertension in patients with pulmonary disease. Chest. 2003;123:222–42.
16. Korn S, Schumann C, Kropf C, Stoiber K, Thielen A, Taube C, et al. Effectiveness of omalizumab in patients 50 years and older with severe persistent allergic asthma. Ann Allergy Asthma Immunol. 2010;105:313–9.
17. Tat T, Cilli A. Evaluation of long-term safety and efficacy of omalizumab in elderly patients with uncontrolled allergic asthma. Ann Allergy Asthma Immunol. 2016;117:546–9.
18. Shimizu Y, Dobashi K, Kusano M, Mori M. Different gastoroesophageal reflux symptoms of middle-aged to elderly asthma and chronic obstructive pulmonary disease (COPD) pateints. J Clin Biochem Nutr. 2012;50:169–75.
19. Mendelsohn A. The effects of reflux on the elderly. The problems with medications and interventions. Otolaryngol Clin North Am. 2018;51:779–87.

20. Ross JA, Yang Y, Song PXK, Clark NM, Baptist AP. Quality of life, health care utilization, and control in older adults with asthma. J Allergy Clin Immunol Pract. 2013;1:157–62.
21. Enright P, McClelland R, Newman A, Gottlieb D, Lebowitz M. Underdiagnosis and under-treatment of asthma in the elderly. Chest. 1999;116:603–13.
22. Bella V, Pedone C, Catalano F, Zito A, Davi E, Palange S, et al. Asthma in the elderly: mortality rate and associated risk factors for mortality. Chest. 2007;132:1175–82.
23. Radenne F, Verkindre C, Tonnel A. Asthma in the elderly. Rev Mal Respir. 2004;21:8s117–25.
24. Connolly M, Yohannes A. The impact of depression in older patients with chronic obstructive pulmonary disease and asthma. Maturitas. 2016;92:9–14.
25. Viera E, Brown E, Raue P. Depression in older adults: screening and referral. J Geriatr Phys Ther. 2014;37:24–30.
26. Harpole L, Williams J, Olsen M, Stechuchak K, Oddone E, Callahan C, et al. Improving depression outcomes in older adults with comorbid medical illness. Gen Hosp Psychiatry. 2005;27:4–12.
27. Bergeron C, Hamid Q. Relationship between asthma and rhinitis: epidemiologic, pathophysiologic, and therapeutic aspects. Allergy Asthma Clin Immunol. 2005;1(2):81–7.
28. Baptist A, Nyenhuis S. Rhinitis in the elderly. Immunol Allergy Clinics N America. 2016;36:343–57.
29. Pinto J, Jeswani S. Rhinitis in the geriatric population. Allergy Asthma Clin Immunology. 2010;6:10.
30. Boulet L, Robitaille C, Deschesnes F, Villeneuve H, Boulay M. Comparative clinical, physiological, and inflammatory characteristics of elderly subjects with or without asthma and young subjects with asthma. Chest. 2017;152:1203–13.
31. Beuther D, Weiss S, Sutherland E. Obesity and asthma. Am J Respir Crit Care Med. 2006;174:112–9.
32. Xu K, Wisivesky J, Martynenko M, Mhango G, Busse P, Wolf M. Assessing the association of obesity and asthma morbidity in older adults. Ann Allergy Asthma Immunol. 2016;117:33–7.
33. Baptist A, Hao W, Karamched K, Kaur B, Carpenter L, Song P. Distinct asthma phenotypes among older adults with asthma. J Allergy Clin Immunol Pract. 2018;6:244–9.
34. Shah R, Yang Y. Health and economic burden of obesity in elderly individuals with asthma in the United States. Popul Health Manag. 2015;18:186–91.
35. Pradeepan S, Garrison G, Dixon A. Obesity in asthma: approaches to treatment. Curr Allergy Asthma Rep. 2013;13:434–42.
36. Melani A. Management of asthma in the elderly patient. Clin Int Aging. 2013;8:913–22.
37. Skloot G, Busse P, Braman S, Kovacs E, Dixon A, Vaz Fragoso CA, et al. An official American Thoracic Society workshop report: evaluation and management of asthma in the elderly. Ann Am Thorac Soc. 2016;11:2064–77.
38. Maher R, Hanlon J, Hajjar E. Clinical consequences of polypharmacy in elderly. Expert Opin Drug Saf. 2014;13:1–11.
39. O'Conor R, Wolf M, Smith S, Martynenko M, Vicencio D, Sano M, et al. Health literacy, cognitive function, proper use, and adherence to inhaled asthma controller medications among older adults with asthma. Chest. 2015;147:2418–25.
40. Kremers H, Larson D, Crowson C, Kremers W, Washington R, Steiner C, et al. Prevalence of total hip and knee replacement in the United States. J Bone Joint Surg Am. 2015;97:1386–97.
41. Chan E, Welsh C. Geriatric respiratory medicine. Chest. 1998;114:1704–33.
42. Peron E, Gray S, Hanlon J. Medication use and functional status decline in older adults: a narrative review. Am J Geriatr Pharmacother. 2011;9:378–91.
43. Burrowa B, Barbee R, Cline M, Knudson R, Lebowitz M. Characteristics of asthma among elderly adults in a sample of the general population. Chest. 1991;100:935–42.
44. Radhakrishna N, Tay T, Hore-Lacy F, Stirling R, Hoy R, Dabscheck E, et al. Validated questionnaires heighten detection of difficult asthma comorbidities. J Asthma. 2017;54:294–9.

Shared Decision-Making and Strategies to Optimize Adherence in Older Asthmatics

8

Don Bukstein and Dennis K. Ledford

> *"At the end of my visit, I may not remember exactly what you said. I may not remember what you did, but I will always remember how you made me feel."*
>
> A Patient

Introduction

Asthma in older adults is a complex and diverse disease with features that vary with the individual patient and with time. As in all aspects of asthma management, it is especially important in older adults to consider the perceptions and beliefs that the patient has about their disease and foster a strong healthcare provider (HCP)/patient partnership to improve nonadherence via true shared decision-making (SDM). Their inevitable functional decline and delayed recovery contribute to the spiral of increasing morbidity and mortality in older asthmatics. To deliver quality healthcare across the continuum of care for this rapidly growing population, effective, well-organized communications as well as adaptive SDM aids are critical.

The transition toward a system of integrated use of improved interactive communication as well as SDM aids for patients with asthma provides a unique

D. Bukstein (✉)
Allergy Asthma Sinus Center, Fitchburg and Milwaukee, Fitchburg, WI, USA

D. K. Ledford
Internal Medicine, James A. Haley VA Hospital, Tampa General Hospital, Moffitt Cancer Center, Advent Health, Tampa, FL, USA
e-mail: dledford@health.usf.edu

© Springer Nature Switzerland AG 2019
T. E. G. Epstein, S. M. Nyenhuis (eds.), *Treatment of Asthma in Older Adults*,
https://doi.org/10.1007/978-3-030-20554-6_8

opportunity for all stakeholders to collaborate with the shared goal of improving asthma care. SDM aids developed for asthma are available from a variety of resources:

- CHEST Foundation
- Allergy & Asthma Network
- American College of Allergy, Asthma & Immunology
- http://asthma.chestnet.org/sdm-tool/

These general SDM aids should be adapted for use in older adult patients. Changes in healthcare delivery in the USA are creating opportunities to achieve this goal with collaborations across healthcare settings. The ideal approach aligns physicians, pharmacists, hospitalists, and other caregivers to make improved communication through SDM more convenient and available to ALL patients.

Asthma has the worst adherence rates among chronic diseases, and this is magnified in the older adult patient [1]. Only 8–13% of patients who fill their initial prescription continue to refill their prescriptions after 1 year [2]; and on average, those who do continue therapy take less than 50% of the prescribed number of doses [3, 4]. Nonadherence can take a variety of forms:

- Erratic, in which the individual misses doses because of forgetfulness or a busy lifestyle
- Inadvertent, in which the individual does not fully understand the specifics of his or her treatment regimen or the need for adherence and thus does not take his or her medication correctly
- Deliberate, in which the individual makes a conscious decision based on perceptions of the burden of illness versus the burden of therapy

Clinicians need to understand the specific form and reasons of therapeutic nonadherence on a case-by-case basis. Improving adherence requires overcoming potential barriers between the patient and the clinician, between the patient and the healthcare system, and between the clinician and the healthcare system (Fig. 8.1) [5].

The objective of this chapter is to provide a discussion of evidence-based, time-efficient strategies that can be adopted by most providers to increase patient adherence using a patient-centered SDM approach that incorporates improved physician communication [6]. These strategies can be implemented at a variety of levels:

- The patient–provider relationship
- The healthcare system
- The group practice (Fig. 8.2)

The objective of these strategies is to develop a system of patient-centered collaborative care, with the goals of enhancing communication and thus improving both adherence and ultimately patient outcomes.

Fig. 8.1 A diagrammatic representation of the multiple interactions necessary to overcome barriers to healthcare

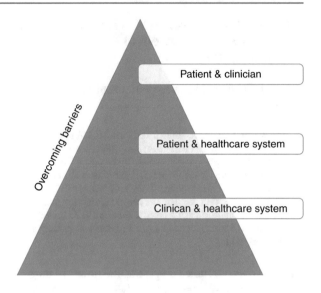

Level of health care system or group practice

- Payment for and development of interactive education
- Making formulary decisions that include adherence factors
- Facilitating depression screening and treatment
- Facilitating communication and SDM with validated decision aids
- Leveraging email, text messages, etc.
- Creating and maintaining system for patient follow-up
- Provider collaboration and training
- Trace medication adherence rates to ED or urgent care visits
- Surveys to identify potential barriers to adherence and optimal patient care
- Patient dashboard as a management tool
- Collecting data on patient medication use and outcomes to identify gaps in care

Level of patient-provider relationship

- Shared decision-making
- Asthma self-management education
- Assessment of patient's perception of asthma control
- Evaluation of patient's health literacy
- Evaluation of factors that are potential barriers to adherence
- OARS motivational interview techniques
- Nonverbal communication techniques
- Using teach-back method to confirm patient understanding
- Develop active partnerships with patient's family
- Monitor patient-provider communication and satisfaction

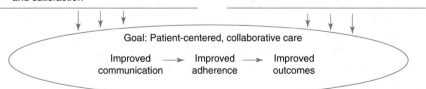

Fig. 8.2 Strategies at the patient–provider level and at the healthcare system/group practice level to promote patient-centered, collaborative care

Turning Nonadherence into Adherence Depends on Establishing a System of Patient-Centered Collaborative Care: Joe's Story

Joe is a 68 year old patient with uncontrolled asthma and poor adherence to his treatment plan.

- Doctor: "So, we're going try this medicine for your poorly controlled asthma; you keep checking how you feel and if daily activities are easier, we can continue with your current medications or add another medicine called 'a biologic.'"
- Patient: "Well, what do we do if the asthma does not get better; if this medicine doesn't work? What are the side effects, cost, and travel requirements?"

My partner told me that she had explained the plan to Joe multiple times and despite reasonable intelligence, he just did not seem to be getting it.

Joe and I were locked in a game of decision-making ping-pong. "What would you do, Doc?" he said.

Such questions trouble caregivers, and often we ping the choice back to patients or "on the one hand, and on the other hand," and Joe begins to realize why Harry Truman joked he wished for a one-handed adviser in the White House.

But the evidence was not clear, and so I directed the choice back to Joe. In our desire to improve patient autonomy, patients are often asked to make hard decisions, to weigh trade-offs, and to wrestle with their own personal values suggesting one path or another. This is particularly true when medical science does not offer a clear answer. Physicians often encourage patients to decide when evidence for one asthma treatment over another is weak. This lack of definitive answers is particularly a problem with older adults, as little evidenced-based data are available for asthma treatment in this age group.

Research suggests that physicians' recommendations powerfully influence how patients weigh their choices, but most patients want to hear options with the confidence their preferences will be considered in the final decision. The greater the uncertainty, the more support they seek, but often the less they receive.

Are Patients Listening as the Clinician Helps Them Navigate the "Gray Zone" of Asthma Care?

It often feels like messages fall on unreceptive ears despite time and effort. Clinicians talk to patients about their asthma, tell them the importance of gaining control, review the risks of uncontrolled asthma, and often include the possibility of remodeling or developing irreversible chronic obstructive pulmonary disease (COPD). The need for compliance with medications is stressed, and a prescription is sent to the pharmacy with refills. When the patient returns for a Focused Asthma Check (see attachment), possibly with an assessment of fractional exhaled nitric oxide (FeNO), the following is discovered:

- The FeNO remains increased.
- The lung function is unchanged or worse.

- Peripheral blood eosinophils are increased or unchanged.
- The Asthma Control Test (ACT) is less than 20.
- Inhaled controller therapy was ideal for a week and then reduced as symptoms improved.

Patients are often overwhelmed with all the information proved, the tasks assigned, the referrals to other professionals, the medicines prescribed, and the lab tests recommended. So it should be no surprise that they end up confused and unsure of what to do next.

How is a more patient-centered system for helping patients achieve their health-related goals constructed? The ideal is for the patient to implement the recommendations provided and to participate in appropriate communication with the healthcare team. This is the challenge of asthma management.

In the brief office/clinic visits, there is almost endless information provided and expectations to do so much in so little time. From clicking boxes in the electronic health record, to filling out forms, to getting prior authorization for medicines, to dealing with insurance companies and pharmacies, the one-to-one communication between the doctor and the patient is often lost.

To accomplish the goals of optimal care, a system is needed that enables health professionals to do what they really want and that is to get back to doctoring.

Printing and providing after-visit summaries have been tried. These have detailed instructions, a list of tests ordered for the patient today, medicines prescribed, a summary plan with instructions for the next few weeks, referrals placed, and more.

Following the patient visit, these detailed instructions often get ignored, the printed copy is filed away or lost, or the email is opened in the patient portal but not accurately answered. Since medical care has evolved into a process unfamiliar to the older adult patient, the clinician often is not speaking the same language or is unaware of the major concern or question. Physicians and other caregivers need to be aware of how language and culture affects patients. It is easier for Joe to understand absolute risks rather than relative risks, i.e., the likelihood that something will happen to Joe rather than the percent change in risk compared to a reference population. Joe was more sensitive to harm than benefits, but the physician in the vignette was emphasizing the effectiveness of therapy. Instead of presenting Joe the choices sequentially, the physician presented them all at once. Joe felt more confident when he was offered a rationale for uncertainty and provided the different therapies, even if the right one for him was not certain. Joe probably worries more about uncommon, terrible events than common, less dramatic outcomes. Physicians on the other hand often struggle more to deal with uncertainty of evidence (information problem) rather than the uncertainty of outcome (prediction problem).

The perfect storm for nonadherence occurs when patient preferences diverge significantly from guideline-based recommendations. In the enthusiasm for guideline adherence, it is often overlooked whether treatment is actually in line with Joe's goals.

Nonadherence in the older adult patient with asthma is not always a matter of forgetting to take one's medication. Most issues of nonadherence are thoughtful

[7–9]. Patients make conscious decisions based on perceptions of the burden of illness (e.g., missed work or school, loss of sleep, chronic symptoms, impaired quality of life, uncertainty or fear, and asthma flares) and the burden of therapy (e.g., reliance on medication, side effects, cost, inconvenience, and needing to schedule appointments). Nonadherence can also be the result of not understanding how to self-manage treatment or the lack of effective communication between the patient and the HCP. Thus, patients must be involved in all aspects of care, from defining the problem to determining therapy [10].

Successful strategies to improve adherence use principles of patient-centered, collaborative care and effective communication. Patient-centered collaborative care identifies patients as experts in their own lives, and clinicians add their medical expertise to what patients know about themselves to create a plan that will help patients achieve their goals [10]. Clinicians can improve patient–provider communication and, in turn medication adherence, with five strategies:

1. Build a relationship.
2. Focus on listening.
3. Collaborate on the treatment plan.
4. Manage time.
5. Implement effective follow-up interventions [6].

In a patient-centered, collaborative system, ideally the patient and physician should have an ongoing relationship and agree upon goals. They also should engage in ongoing monitoring and SDM. Both the patient and clinician should understand the heterogeneity of response and expect the possibility of nonresponse and heightened susceptibility to adverse effects.

Strategies to Improve Adherence in the Older Adult Patient

Communication and SDM

Better communication and SDM can improve adherence, thus leading to improved asthma outcomes [11, 12]. Better communication first involves the clinician identifying nonadherence and its underlying cause [13]. The provider can then emphasize the value of the treatment regimen and elicit the patient's feelings about his or her ability to follow the regimen. Communication also entails providing simple and clear instructions and simplifying the regimen as much as possible, and customizing the regimen in accordance with the patient's wishes. Obtaining help from family members, friends, and community services and reinforcing desirable behavior are also part of the communication process.

A Personal and Empathetic Approach

Better communication is important when addressing the underlying intuitions that drive patient preferences. Physician responses to patient reactions vary, and physicians may be concerned that resisting patient desires may decrease satisfaction. Physicians can also be vulnerable to anticipated regret triggered by recall of patient's perceptions in past treatment scenarios with poor outcomes.

Lack of Proper Communication

Ineffective communication can lead to frustration in both the older adult and their caregiver, when applicable. Some of the barriers are due to their reduced hearing capacity or inability to express their thoughts clearly. Since communication involves a clear exchange of information involving two parties, a gap exists when one or both of the parties has barriers to full functioning. The ability to identify the source of the problem will consequently determine the steps the care provider needs to take in order to resolve them. Solutions can be as simple as finding an alternative means to communicate outside of verbal signals, or as intricate as medical treatment to improve the physical limitation.

There are various reasons why older adults lose their ability to communicate properly. Some of the most common reasons are:

- Failing hearing – When people age, they undergo anatomical changes. Reduced hearing capacity is a natural effect involved with the natural aging process. When an older adult lacks proper hearing capacity, they do not recognize when someone is talking or do not hear complete sentences nor clearly understand the information being relayed. Often the older patient is either unaware of the communication lapse or embarrassed to request that statements be repeated. Speech discrimination may be impaired much more than tone perception. There are improved hearing aids available to help address this issue, but the devices are usually expensive. Another option is to record the clinical visit or record only the recommendations so that they can be reviewed later in a less stressful environment by the patient and/or family members.
- Vision problems or failing eyesight – Another natural effect of aging is reduced eyesight. Therefore, older people have difficulty reading written communication. The effects of poor eyesight can be reduced by using alternative communication schemes, larger-print material, or encouragement of the use of corrective lenses.
- Effect of medications – This cause for communication problems is potentially reversible. Adverse effects of many common medications in older adults include fatigue or reduced cognitive function. Polypharmacy, impaired drug metabolism, and complex drug interactions complicate the identification of the culprit drug.
- Structural or neurological damage – This situation is often caused by other diseases such as intracranial mass lesions, Alzheimer's disease, Parkinson's disease, or cerebral vascular accidents. Most of these conditions produce permanent impairment, but there are a few coping mechanisms and strategies that can be provided for patients so that they are able to communicate effectively. Lack of recognition of these neurologic conditions will complicate and limit the effectiveness of any adjustment.

Communication problems involved in caring for older adults need to be identified as quickly as possible to enable accommodation strategies. A few principles that may be helpful include:

- Understand the two-way process of communication – Effective communication involves a clear exchange of information between the speaker and hearer; therefore both have to cooperate.
- Make communication adjustments – The clinician should be sensitive and aware of potential problems with communication and take action. The communication pattern cannot be adjusted until the source of the problem is identified.

Nonverbal Communication and Aids

Once the source of the communication problem has been determined, the effects can be mitigated by utilizing devices and aids designed specifically to foster better communication. Strategies include:

- Eyeglasses and hearing aids – These are recommended for older adults who are suffering from a decline in eyesight and hearing.
- Large-print reading material or graphics – Using written material or pictures instead of spoken communication may help prevent frustration. In addition, enduring materials may be utilized by family and caregivers.
- Enlisting the assistance of family and caregivers – Requesting the presence of family and caregivers, with the approval of the patient, may also be an effective strategy to improve communication.

Scheduled and Monitored Follow-Up

Another component of patient-centered, collaborative care involves creating and maintaining a system for follow-up. This is easier to do in integrated systems. Such a system needs to include specialty-controlled triage that focuses on high-risk populations and involves modern tools for dealing with depression and adherence. The primary care provider then has limited, straightforward disease management skills and uses technology to assist at point of service. Such a system teaches and fosters behavioral medicine and provides a system that facilitates and rewards. Healthcare providers then monitor outcomes and redirect patients, using technology to monitor and advise.

Triggers to Encourage Family and Friends to Seek Assistance for the Patient

When all the procedures indicated above have been utilized and there are still communication problems, then it may be time to seek professional help. Asking for professional help must be done during the following circumstances:

- An older asthmatic adult has difficulty speaking, understanding, or communicating.
- An older person exhibits unusual vocalization that is neither caused by cold nor flu.
- Speech becomes incomprehensible.
- An older person fails to respond consistently.

Positive Communication Strategies

Communication is a two-way street. A personal and empathetic approach to asking questions about asthma self-management is recommended. When given the opportunity to raise questions and reveal beliefs, older patients may acknowledge that they dislike the idea of taking a specific medication. It is best practice to approach the patient with a mix of closed- and open-ended questions that are nonjudgmental. SDM will also make the patient feel more comfortable and willing to discuss any concerns and issues that they might have. Adopting a SDM approach will allow them to feel more empowered and also help with the development of a collaborative, long-term, personalized management plan which will improve adherence [11].

Strategies for SDM include:

1. *Listening skills*

   The HCP who is a sincere, attentive listener is the cornerstone of effective communication. Studies show that the average physician interrupts their patient within 10–20 seconds of the initiation of conversation. Of course, physicians have to remain focused due to time constraints, but 20 seconds is not sufficient for an important story.

2. *Interpersonal skills with patients and colleagues*

   Awareness of image portrayed during conversation is frequently lacking, and this is also true of HCPs. The focus on disease identification and technical details may detract from the human connection. Very subtle verbal and nonverbal behaviors will determine on a psychological level whether people connect especially in a professional situation. There are a myriad of factors including tone of voice, acknowledgement of what the other person is saying, and facial expression. Most physicians can easily learn techniques to improve these skills.

3. *Empathy and emotional intelligence*

   Empathy is a trait that is intrinsically linked to many communication skills, especially listening. Emotional intelligence is the capability to recognize both your own and others' emotions and to modify your behavior based upon this insight. Healthcare, being based upon a unique, personal interaction, benefits from the clinician possessing a high level of emotional intelligence. This will greatly enable the healthcare profession to exhibit more compassion – a crucial aspect of being an effective clinician. This attribute is essential for productive communication and SDM, with or without SDM aids, in all age groups but particularly with the older adult patient.

Shared Decision-Making (SDM)

The preceding discussion highlights aspects of SDM. SDM improves asthma therapy adherence in all age groups but particularly in older adults. SDM is a process based on mutual respect and partnership that aims to help patients receive the care they prefer. SDM involves four key elements in the exchange between the patient and the HCP.

- Sharing of relevant information
- Expression of treatment preferences
- Deliberation of the options
- Agreement on the treatment plan [11]·

SDM can be facilitated with decisional aids. Two aids for SDM in asthma management have recently been developed (asthma.chestnet.org and the American College of Allergy Asthma and Immunology (ACAAI) or Allergy Asthma Network web sites). Additional examples of SDM aids are available from the Ottawa Hospital Research Institute (https://decisionaid.ohri.ca/). These decision aids and risk pictographs are more useful for uncertainty of outcomes than for uncertainty of evidence; the former is generally of greater importance to the patient.

Older asthmatics often need assistance in systematically identifying what is important to them and in developing goals and preferences. This awareness assists the older adult patient in the evaluation of their options. The University of California, San Francisco, for example, coaches patients through a decision-making process via a team of paid and unpaid interns called the Patient Support Corps [14]. This program utilizes SDM processes by contacting patients prior to visits. The pre-visit coaching utilizes decision aids to better educate patients about treatment options and outcomes and communication aids to enhance the information exchange during the visit. Survey data collected over 3 years confirmed the effectiveness of the SDM intervention. The costs of the program were estimated to be $145,000/year with the utilization of paid students for the coaching. This expenditure connected 4500 patients and 22 staff physicians and dozens of residents, fellows, and nurses in a SDM process during 3 years in a specialty breast clinic [11, 15].

Asthma Self-Management Education

Asthma self-management education is essential for providing patients with the skills necessary to control asthma and improve outcomes [16]. Only 1 of 3 older adult asthmatic patients receives an Asthma Action Plan, and almost none receive a change of lifestyle plan. Most older asthmatic patients are not provided education on peak-flow assessment or recognition of signs and symptoms of asthma, and nearly 50% of patients do not receive education on environmental control measures [17]. The National Asthma Education and Prevention Program

	Assessment questions	Information and skills

Initial visit	• "What worries you most about your asthma?"
	• "What do you want to accomplish at this visit?"
	• "What do you want to be able to do that you can't do now because of your asthma?"
	• "What do you expect from treatment?"
	• "What medicines have you tried?"
	• "Are there things in your environment that make your asthma worse?"
		Teach in simple language
		• What is asthma? Asthma is a chronic lung disease. The airways are very sensitive. They become inflamed and narrow, and breathing becomes difficult.
		• The definition of asthma control: few daytime symptoms, no nighttime awakenings due to asthma, able to engage in normal activities normal lung function
		• Asthma treatments: 2 types of medicines are needed:
		  • Long-term control: medications that prevent symptoms, often by reducing inflammation
		  • Quick relief: short-acting bronchodilator relaxes muscles around airways
		• Tell patient to bring all medications to every appointment
		• Tell patient when to seek medical advice and provide appropriate telephone number
		Teach and demonstrate
		• Correct inhaler and spacer or VHC technique and check performance
		• Self-monitoring skills that are tied to a written action plan:
		  • Recognize intensity and frequency of asthma symptoms
		  • Review the signs of deterioration and the need to reevaluate therapy:
		    • Waking at night or early morning with asthma
		    • Increased medication use
		    • Decreased activity tolerance
		• Use of a written asthma action plan that includes instructions for daily management and for recognizing and handling worsening asthma

1st follow-up visit	• Ask relevant questions from previous visit • "What medications are you taking?" • "How and when are you taking them?" • "What problems have you had using your medications?" • "Please show me how you use your inhaled medications."	**Teach in simple language** • Use of 2 types of medications • Remind patient to bring all medications and peak flow monitor, if using, to every appointment for review • Self-assessment of asthma control using symptoms and/or peak flow as a guide **Teach or review and demonstrate** • Use of written asthma action plan; review and adjust as needed • Peak flow monitoring if indicated • Correct inhaler and spacer or VHC technique

2nd follow-up visit	• Ask relevant questions from previous visit
	• "Have you noticed anything in your home, work, or school that makes your asthma worse?"
	• "Describe for me how you know when to call your doctor or go to the hospital for asthma care."
	• "What questions do you have about the asthma action plan? Can we make it easier?"
	• "Are your medications causing you any problems?"
	• "Have you noticed anything in your environment that makes your asthma worse?"
	• "Have you missed any of your medications?"
		Teach in simple language
		• Self-assessment of asthma control using symptoms and/or peak flow as a guide
		• Relevant environmental control/avoidance strategies
		  • How to identify home, work, or school exposures that can cause or worsen asthma
		  • How to control house-dust mites and animal exposures, if applicable
		  • How to avoid cigarette smoke (active and passive)
		• Review all medications
		Teach or review and demonstrate
		• Correct inhaler and spacer or VHC technique
		• Peak flow monitoring if indicated
		• Use of written asthma action plan; review and adjust as needed
		• Confirm that patient knows what to do if asthma gets worse

All subsequent visits	• Ask relevant questions from previous visit
	• "How have you tried to control things that make your asthma worse?"
	• "Please show me how you use your inhaled medication."
		Teach in simple language
		• Review and reinforce all
		  • Educational messages
		  • Environmental control strategies at home, work, or school
		  • Medications
		  • Self-assessment of asthma control, using symptoms and/ or peak flow as a guide
		Teach or review and demonstrate
		• Correct inhaler and spacer or VHC technique
		• Peak flow monitoring if indicated
		• Use of written asthma action plan; review and adjust as needed
		• Confirm that patient knows what to do if asthma gets worse

Fig. 8.3 Recommended asthma education during patient care visits. Adapted from the National Asthma Education and Prevention Program, Third Expert Panel on the Diagnosis and Management of Asthma. Expert Panel Report 3: Guidelines for the Diagnosis and Management of Asthma. Bethesda (MD): National Heart, Lung, and Blood Institute (US); 2007 Aug. Section 3, Component 2: Education for a Partnership in Asthma Care. Available from: https://www.ncbi.nlm.nih.gov/books/NBK7239/ [16]

(NAEPP) Guidelines for the Diagnosis and Management of Asthma recommends that education is integrated into all aspects of asthma care (Fig. 8.3) [16]. That being said, most patients are not asked about control. Asthma self-management, like clinician-based asthma guideline management, depends entirely on accurate assessments of control status merged with the individual goals of therapy. Continuous education and SDM are needed from diagnosis to follow-up care, and education includes repetition and reinforcement. Such an approach involves all members of the healthcare team. Benefits of self-management education are:

- Reduction in urgent care visits and hospitalizations
- Reduction of asthma-related healthcare costs
- Improvement in health status
- Reduction in symptoms
- Reduction of limitations on activity
- Improvement of quality of life
- Enhancement of control of asthma
- Improvement in medication adherence [16]

Essential elements for asthma self-management include individually tailored, asthma self-management education with key messages and goals [16]. Patients should be trained to self-monitor symptoms, and they should have written asthma action plans or lifestyle plans. An Asthma Report Card (ARC), which is for the patient and the physician, can be used to regularly review a patient's asthma control. The ARC reflects a continuous cycle of assessment, treatment, and review (Fig. 8.4) [18]. Essential elements also include an active partnership with the patient and family and encouragement of adherence via SDM with decisional aids.

Key educational messages for patients should include basic facts about asthma, what defines well-controlled asthma, and the patient's current level of control [16]. The message should also include information on how medications play a role in asthma management. Patient education also needs to include demonstration of skills, including using a spacer or valved holding chamber, as well as instruction in self-monitoring. In addition, the educational message should specify when and how

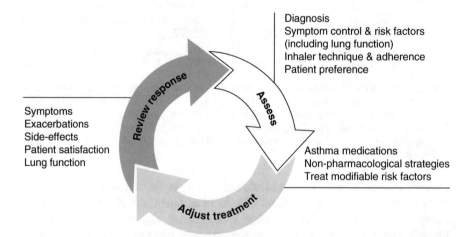

Fig. 8.4 The control-based asthma management cycle that incorporates assessment, treatment, and review. Republished with permission from the Global Initiative for Asthma (GINA) Global Strategy for Asthma Management and Prevention [18]

to handle signs and symptoms of worsening asthma and when and where to seek care. The patient should also learn about environmental exposure control measures, the role of allergen immunotherapy, value of smoking cessation at any age, and the importance of vaccinations including annual influenza, pertussis, and pneumococcal immunization.

Asthma self-management education can and should occur at multiple coordinated points of care and be clinic- or office-based, pharmacy-based, hospital-based, community-based, and home-based with consistent messaging [16]. Furthermore, technologies that are already part of the patient's daily life such as the internet and mobile devices can be used to engage patients. Potential benefits include better patient–provider communication, an informed provider between visits, continual monitoring of asthma status, and early detection of asthma exacerbation. However, such technologies may not be appropriate for all patients, and their use depends on computer and health literacies, access, and patient preferences. The older adult patient may be uncomfortable with the use of web-based and other electronic resources.

NAEPP guidelines recommend monitoring at each visit [16]. At each visit, the clinician should assess the patient's adherence to the regimen, inhaler technique (with documentation), side effects of medications using SDM, patient satisfaction with asthma control via the Asthma Report Card or equivalent, and patient satisfaction with a quality of care survey. Accomplishing all, or even most, of these in a brief visit is a challenge, demonstrating the need for regular outpatient visits to obtain this information. A negative attitude concerning medications or self-management is a risk factor for severe exacerbations.

Clinicians should consider education to enhance knowledge and skills. Asthma providers should consider easy-to-understand, interactive education in asthma care and participating in programs to enhance skills in patient communication [16]. Clinicians may also wish to consider developing and using clinical pathways for the management of acute asthma. Also recommended are developing, implementing, and evaluating system-based interventions to support clinical decision-making and quality care for asthma. These suggestions are not unique to care of the older asthmatic, but the increased risk and healthcare utilization in the older age group increase the importance of these options.

Assessments to Be Made by the Clinician

As part of the asthma self-management education process, the provider should assess the patient's perception of their asthma control, the patient's health literacy, and other factors that are potential barriers to asthma control. In patient-centered, collaborative care, the clinician has the responsibility to get the patient's perception of his or her illness (PPI). This includes asking patients what bothers them about their asthma and whether they think they need better asthma control. Studies show that patients often believe that their asthma is under good control, when in fact the occurrence of multiple asthma exacerbations or the use of albuterol both at daytime and nighttime shows that the asthma is not under good control [19, 20]. Patients might set the bar too low. The clinician should also ask patients what they are looking for from their therapies. On the other hand, in the older adult patient, achieving optimal asthma control may be less important than allowing a reasonable quality of life and activity level. The goal of asthma care is modified by the PPI and expectations.

The clinician also needs to evaluate the patient's health literacy, or the ability to read, understand, and act on healthcare information [21]. Health literacy affects people's ability to use SDM, navigate the healthcare system, share personal information such as health histories with providers, engage in self-care and chronic disease management, and understand mathematical concepts such as probability and risk [22]. Health literacy is a strong predictor of a person's health – more so than age, income, employment status, education level, and race [23]. Providers should assess patients' health literacy and look for cues of limited health literacy, such as glancing over the page without focusing on the words, making errors regarding medication, answering incorrectly when questioned about what they have read, and using excuses such as "I forgot my glasses" [24].

Providers can use a variety of techniques to improve patients' health literacy via proactive care management [25]. These include ordering information from the most to least important, slowing down, speaking slowly, and spending adequate additional time with each patient. These are particularly important in older adults and may require increasing staff responsibilities to do this work. Providers should also use plain, nonmedical language and frame instructions using illustrative anecdotes, drawings, pictures, videos, tables, and graphs. Using numbers instead of percentages and simplifying other numeric concepts whenever possible are other effective strategies. Clinicians should ensure that medication-dosing instructions are clear. Another technique is limiting the amount of information and then repeating it. Providers can also use a teach-back or "show me" approach to confirm understanding, encourage questions, and create a shame-free environment. This is especially important in medication management, as it is a very effective assessment technique for the patient to demonstrate the use of their inhaler or describe the differences in the inhalers.

The synchronized prescription renewal or refill is another easy way to improve adherence while decreasing physician and staff time refilling chronic medications. At a dedicated annual comprehensive care visit, renew all medications for chronic illness for the maximum duration allowed by state law. Include instructions for the pharmacy on all prescription modifications and renewals as applicable (e.g., "Do not fill until patient calls" or "Place on hold"). Take the opportunity to renew all of the patient's prescriptions for chronic conditions when you receive a prescription renewal request. Any visit is a good time to renew all medications for chronic illness because during this visit the patient's medical history is thoroughly reviewed, including past and present conditions and medications. During this visit all medications for chronic illness should be renewed for the maximum duration (12–15 months in most states). When a patient has received prescriptions for their chronic conditions for the upcoming year, they will not need to call the office for refills, and they will not have any unanticipated gaps in medication adherence.

Most Nonadherence is **Intentional**

Fear	Cost	Misunderstanding	Too many medications
Potential side effects or side effects they had previously with the same or a similar medication; saw side effects in friend/family member taking similar medication	Patients may not fill medications in the first place or ration what they do fill to extend their supply	Patients may not understand the need for the medicine, the nature of side effects or the expected time it will take to see results	The greater the number of different medicines prescribed and the higher the dosing frequency, the more likely a patient is to be nonadherent

Lack of symptoms	Worry	Depression	Mistrust
Patients who don't feel any differently when they start or stop their medicine may see no reason to take it	Concerns about becoming dependent on a medicine also leads to nonadherence	Patients who are depressed are less likely to take their medications as prescribed	Patients may be suspicious of their doctor's motives for prescribing certain medications (eg, news of pharmaceutical companies influencing physician prescribing patterns)

AMA. Practice transformation series: Medication adherence. 2015

Fig. 8.5 Top reasons for intentional nonadherence. Most nonadherences are intentional. Patients make a rational decision not to take their medicine based on their knowledge, experience, and beliefs. From AMA, Practice transformation series: Medication adherence. 2015 https://edhub. ama-assn.org/steps-forward/module/2702595#section-201978139

Finally, the clinician should assess other factors that could be potential barriers to adherence (Fig. 8.5). Socioeconomic factors include poverty, illiteracy, low educational achievement, unemployment, insufficient social support, transportation issues, excessive medication and treatment costs, and environmental factors. Health system factors include problems with patient–provider relationships, inadequate local health services, insufficient reimbursement from health insurance, insufficient knowledge and training for healthcare providers on managing chronic diseases, lack of incentives and feedback on performance, inconsistent clinical staff due to turn over or rotations of staff, and inadequate system emphasis and support for patient education. Condition-related factors include symptom burden, frailty, activity limitation, availability of effective treatments, and the influence of comorbidities. Therapy-related factors include polypharmacy and treatment complexity, previous failures with therapy, frequent changes in treatment, lack of perceived beneficial effects, and side effects. Patient-related factors include self-efficacy, cognitive ability, concern over side effects, cosmetic concerns, motivation, attitudes, awareness of respiratory status, cultural beliefs and perceptions, and psychological issues. In particular, clinicians should assess patients for anxiety and depression, since these conditions decrease adherence [26–31].

Tips and Techniques for the Clinician

Clinicians have several available techniques to facilitate communication in order to improve adherence. The Scoped technique was previously discussed. Another approach is the OARS motivational interview, which entails asking open-ended questions (O), affirming what the patient says (A), using reflective listening (R), and summarizing back to the patient what he or she has been saying (S) [32]. In addition, clinicians can employ key strategies such as a congenial demeanor, which includes friendliness, humor, and attentiveness, and patience to allow the patient to express his or her goals, beliefs, and concerns. Empathy, reassurance, and prompt handling of any concerns are also beneficial strategies. Offering encouragement and praise, giving appropriate and personalized information, and providing feedback and review also facilitate good communication.

Other techniques include asking a second person, such as a nurse or family member, to repeat the main messages to the patient and paying attention to nonverbal communication by the patient, such as poor eye contact. Providers should make patients feel comfortable about asking questions. Finally, clinician should limit their time using a computer while talking to a patient. A recent study showed that patients with limited proficiency in English and limited health literacy in safety-net clinics had lower patient satisfaction when clinicians frequently used their computers during office visits, thus inhibiting engagement and missing openings for deeper connections with their patients [33]. Unfortunately, the reality of current utilization of electronic healthcare records usurps physician time and focus away from the patient and to the computer screen. This situation may not be readily changed, but physician awareness of this issue may provide opportunities to modify the patient–physician interaction.

To improve communication, clinicians should also develop an active partnership with the patient's family and/or caregivers [16]. This strategy also entails tailoring the asthma self-management, teaching approach to the needs of each situation, while maintaining sensitivity to cultural beliefs and ethnocultural practices. Cultural competency is important in this context. A "placed-based" organizing framework, reflecting five key areas of social determinates of health (SDOH), was developed by Healthy People 2020. They are:

1. Economic stability
2. Education
3. Social and community context (old and young working together)
4. Health and healthcare access at low cost
5. Neighborhood and built environment as well as easy access to physician and pharmacy

Monitoring Patient–Provider Communication and Satisfaction

Another key element to improving adherence is monitoring patient–provider communication and satisfaction. One approach is to have the patient fill out a questionnaire before the visit [16]. Example questions include:

- "What questions have you had about your asthma daily self-management plan and action plan?"
- "What problems have you had following the daily self-management plan or action plan?"
- "How do you feel about making your own decisions about therapy?"

- "Has anything prevented you from getting the treatment you need for your asthma from me or anyone else?"
- "Have the costs of your asthma treatment interfered with your ability to get asthma care?"
- "How satisfied are you with your asthma care?"
- "How can we improve your asthma care?"

Strategies at the Healthcare System or Group Practice Level

Systems approach to the older adult asthma patient is an approach that aligns physicians, pharmacists, hospitalists, ED physicians, and other caregivers to make SDM more convenient and available to all patients. Advantages are:

1. Sharing resources from well-developed SDM programs can help with education on improved policies, practice, and knowledge to increase utilization of aids and assist in staff training to improve efficiency.
2. Sharing knowledge on SDM and aids especially about unique populations like older adult is important. SDM delivery and coordination can lead to better understanding of challenges and opportunities with more widespread use of SDM aids for asthma treatment.
3. Clinical algorithms can lead to wider use of SDM and compensation to healthcare providers doing SDM.

Since asthma in older adults remains a major cause of ED visits and hospitalizations, meaningful collaborations with medical systems (asthma COPD overlap, Managed care, Medicaid) have the potential for improving care, patient satisfaction, and adherence. These collaborations may result in fewer admissions, reduced direct and indirect asthma costs, and patient activation for better self-management. Consultations are an opportunity for HCPs and the older patient to meet and work together in a SDM process to optimize asthma management and ensure that an optimal lifestyle-care plan is in place.

The healthcare system can also encourage adherence by promoting, providing, and paying for education that is interactive, making formulary decisions that include adherence factors, using copays to promote effective care, facilitating depression screening and treatment, improving access to skilled clinicians, and facilitating communication and SDM with validated decisional aids.

Additional strategies that HCPs can implement include creating a team-based approach to work collaboratively with patients and their caregivers to accomplish shared goals within and across settings for coordinated, high-quality care [34]. This approach establishes clear roles, mutual trust, and effective communication among team members. Monthly meetings within a group practice to present difficult cases and receive feedback are another strategy. HCPs can use a patient dashboard as a management tool for both patients and physicians. The dashboard displays key data and trends in the Asthma Report Card or equivalent, including the patient's current status and activity over time. HCPs can use this tool to compare an individual patient to other patients in the group, the region, or the nation. They can also use dashboards to determine whether they are meeting internal targets among peers or external targets such as NAEPP guidelines. Furthermore, patients can view their diagnosis, treatment, and status and access a patient portal for education and group visits.

As part of team-based care, HCPs might want to consider using charts so that HCPs can record when specific tasks involved in the long-term management of asthma were performed and who performed the task. Tasks might include teaching the patient to monitor for and avoid triggers, checking medication adherence, distributing educational tools, and reaching out to the patient after an appointment. HCPs can also encourage adherence by leveraging email and SMS text messages, which are used as healthcare reminders in a variety of chronic diseases [35–40].

Furthermore, a group practice or healthcare system can implement several action items. Group practices and healthcare systems should continually assess and strive for an atmosphere that fosters patient-centric care. They can trace medication adherence rates to emergency department or urgent care visits. Patient and provider surveys can be used to identify potential barriers to adherence and to optimal patient care. HCPs should also institute programs that encourage adherence, promote patient education that provides pathways to adherence, and implement guidelines for managing nonadherence.

Better communication and adherence is about patient engagement. Interactions between patients and their HCPs at all levels contribute to the patient's experience both positively and negatively. These interactions ultimately affect communication and adherence. Changes in healthcare delivery, financing, technology, and especially electronic medical records (EMRs) have created both opportunities and challenges [41–45]. This means that clinicians and systems must begin to better engage their patients with enhanced collaboration. Bloomrosen and Sennett [46] identify several strategies for patient engagement for incorporating patient-reported and patient-generated data, assessing patients' preferences, and informing patient–HCP communications. For example, to incorporate patient-reported and patient-generated data, HCPs might consider leveraging patient engagement work undertaken by patient and disease advocacy groups and specialty societies. A strategy for assessing patients' preferences includes confirming patient values, needs, and goals as part of SDM. To inform patient–provider communications, one option is to form patient advisory boards or councils to provide input, feedback, and opinions.

Conclusions

Adherence to an individual's treatment regimen should be assessed and encouraged at every visit. Figure 8.6 provides a checklist of strategies for this. HCPs should use effective techniques to promote open communication and begin each visit by asking about the patient's concerns and goals. They should also ask specifically about any concerns about medications or treatment. Polypharmacy, with the inherent risk for drug interaction and with increased cost, is a major challenge in treating asthma in

Assess and encourage adherence during all asthma visits	
Use effective techniques to promote open communication	✓
Begin each visit by asking about the patient's concerns and goals	✓
Ask specifically about any concerns about medications/treatment	✓
Assess patient's perception of their asthma severity and how well it is controlled	✓
Assess patient's level of social support; encourage family involvement	✓
Assess levels of stress, family disruption, anxiety, and depression associated with asthma and its management	✓
Assess patient's ability to adhere to the written action plan	✓

Fig. 8.6 Tips for improving adherence adapted from the National Asthma Education and Prevention Program Guidelines for the Diagnosis and Management of Asthma [16]

older adults. HCPs should assess the patient's perception of their asthma severity and control as well as the patient's level of stress, family disruption, anxiety, and depression. Especially in older adults, it is important to identify the patient's perception of need or goals and not simply rely upon guideline-based goals of control and optimal lung function. The older asthmatic may prefer less medications and a lower lung function, as long as functional status is acceptable and exacerbation risk is low. Finally, HCPs should assess the patient's ability to adhere to the written action plan and simplify the regimen if possible.

Improving patient–HCP communication is key to improving adherence, thus reducing poor health outcomes and significant indirect and direct healthcare costs. Communication and involvement of the patient are ways to improve adherence in currently nonadherent patients, reinforce the benefits of adherence in currently adherent patients, and minimize the risk of nonadherence in new patients. The first step in effective patient–provider communication is to break down barriers using SDM decisional aids [47].

In addition, clinicians should assess the patient's health literacy, anxiety, confusion, language and cultural issues, medication adherence, and support system. Another strategy to improve communication is exploring options to motivate and improve self-management. Finally, clinicians need to evaluate whether their practice is user-friendly and implement improvements where possible. By implementing a variety of evidence-based approaches to create patient-centered, collaborative care, HCPs can improve patient–HCP communication, thus improving adherence and patient outcomes. Future directions should focus on research and development of new, cost-effective innovative educational interventions that use technology to assist education and psychological support strategies to encourage learning, motivation, self-efficacy, and behavior change. These changes, along with SDM strategies, are likely to improve healthcare providers' engagement with patients and ultimately improve medication adherence.

Acknowledgments The authors sincerely thank Sally Sochessler for her assistance and advisement.

Financial Disclosures Dr. Bukstein declares that he has received honoraria as a speaker for AstraZeneca, Circassia, Genentech, ALK, Merck, Novartis, and Teva.

Dr. Dennis Ledford provided consultation services for AstraZeneca and Genentech; received research support paid to institution from AstraZeneca and Genentech; served as a member of speaker bureau for AstraZeneca, Boehringer Ingelheim, Genentech/Roche, Novartis, and Teva; and participated in legal reviews for cases of sudden asthma death, immunotherapy and adverse reactions, drug allergy, and indoor fungal exposure.

Funder Statement The work for this article was not funded.

References

1. Vanelli M, Adler S, Vermilyea J. Moving beyond market share. In Vivo: The Business and Medicine Report. 2002;(Part 3):67–74. https://www.pharmamedtechbi.com/Publications/IN-VIVO/20/3/Moving-Beyond-Market-Share
2. Borrelli B, Riekert KA, Weinstein A, Rathier L. Brief motivational interviewing as a clinical strategy to promote asthma medication adherence. J Allergy Clin Immunol. 2007;120(5):1023–30.
3. Bender BG. Advancing the science of adherence measurement: implications for the clinician. J Allergy Clin Immunol Pract. 2013;1(1):92–3.
4. Vik SA, Maxwell CJ, Hogan DB. Measurement, correlates, and health outcomes of medication adherence among seniors. Ann Pharmacother. 2004;38(2):303–12.
5. Bukstein D, Luskin AT, Farrar JR. The reality of adherence to rhinitis treatment: identifying and overcoming the barriers. Allergy Asthma Proc. 2011;32(4):265–71.
6. Bender BG. Promoting adherence and effective self-management in patients with asthma. In: Leung DY, Szefler SJ, Bonilla FA, Akdis CA, Sampson H, editors. Pediatric allergy: principles and practice. 3rd ed. Edinburgh: Elsevier; 2016. p. 354–359.e352.
7. Bender B, Milgrom H, Rand C, Ackerson L. Psychological factors associated with medication nonadherence in asthmatic children. J Asthma. 1998;35(4):347–53.
8. Little P, Everitt H, Williamson I, et al. Preferences of patients for patient centred approach to consultation in primary care: observational study. BMJ. 2001;322(7284):468–72.
9. McKinstry B. Do patients wish to be involved in decision making in the consultation? A cross sectional survey with video vignettes. BMJ. 2000;321(7265):867–71.
10. Bodenheimer T, Lorig K, Holman H, Grumbach K. Patient self-management of chronic disease in primary care. JAMA. 2002;288(19):2469–75.
11. Wilson SR, Strub P, Buist AS, et al. Shared treatment decision making improves adherence and outcomes in poorly controlled asthma. Am J Respir Crit Care Med. 2010;181(6):566–77.
12. Rivera-Spoljaric K, Halley M, Wilson SR. Shared clinician-patient decision-making about treatment of pediatric asthma: what do we know and how can we use it? Curr Opin Allergy Clin Immunol. 2014;14(2):161–7.
13. Osterberg L, Blaschke T. Adherence to medication. N Engl J Med. 2005;353(5):487–97.
14. Belkora J, Volz S, Loth M, Teng A, et al. Coaching patients in the use of decision and communication aids: RE-AIM evaluation of a patient support program. BMC Health Serv Res. 2015;15:209.

15. Veroff D, Marr A, Wennberg DE. Enhanced support for shared decision making reduced costs of care for patients with preference-sensitive conditions. Health Aff. 2013;32(2):285–93.
16. National Asthma Education and Prevention Program. Expert panel report 3: guidelines for the diagnosis and management of asthma. Bethesda: National Heart, Lung, and Blood Institute (US); 2007.
17. Office of Disease Prevention and Health Promotion. 2020 Topics and objectives: respiratory diseases. Healthy People 2020; 2014. http://www.healthypeople.gov/2020/topics-objectives/topic/respiratory-diseases/objectives#5182
18. Global Initiative for Asthma (GINA). Global strategy for asthma management and prevention; April 2015. http://www.ginasthma.org/local/uploads/files/GINA_Report_2015_Aug11.pdf
19. Nathan RA, Thompson PJ, Price D, et al. Taking aim at asthma around the world: global results of the asthma insight and management survey in the Asia-Pacific Region, Latin America, Europe, Canada, and the United States. J Allergy Clin Immunol Pract. 2015;3(5):734–742 e735.
20. Kendrick AH, Higgs CM, Whitfield MJ, Laszlo G. Accuracy of perception of severity of asthma: patients treated in general practice. BMJ. 1993;307(6901):422–4.
21. Fact sheet #1: What is health literacy? Center for Health Care Strategies, Inc; October 2013. http://www.chcs.org/media/What_is_Health_Literacy.pdf.
22. Quick guide to health literacy. U.S. Department of Health and Human Services, Office of Disease Prevention and Health Promotion. http://health.gov/communication/literacy/quickguide/Quickguide.pdf
23. Health literacy. National Network of Libraries of Medicine; 5 Aug 2014. http://nnlm.gov/outreach/consumer/hlthlit.html
24. Cornett S. Assessing and addressing health literacy. Online J Issues Nurs. 2009;14(3). http://www.nursingworld.org/MainMenuCategories/ANAMarketplace/ANAPeriodicals/OJIN/TableofContents/Vol142009/No3Sept09/Assessing-Health-Literacy-.html
25. Weiss BD. Health literacy and patient safety: help patients understand. Manual for clinicians. 2nd ed. Florida State University College of Medicine. http://med.fsu.edu/userFiles/file/ahec_health_clinicians_manual.pdf. May 2007.
26. Bender BG. Risk taking, depression, adherence, and symptom control in adolescents and young adults with asthma. Am J Respir Crit Care Med. 2006;173(9):953–7.
27. Barnes CB, Ulrik CS. Asthma and adherence to inhaled corticosteroids: current status and future perspectives. Respir Care. 2015;60(3):455–68.
28. Rosenkranz MA, Busse WW, Sheridan JF, Crisafi GM, Davidson RJ. Are there neurophenotypes for asthma? Functional brain imaging of the interaction between emotion and inflammation in asthma. PLoS One. 2012;7(8):e40921.
29. Thomas M, Bruton A, Moffat M, Cleland J. Asthma and psychological dysfunction. Prim Care Respir J. 2011;20(3):250–6.
30. Spinhoven P, van Peski-Oosterbaan AS, Van der Does AJ, Willems LN, Sterk PJ. Association of anxiety with perception of histamine induced bronchoconstriction in patients with asthma. Thorax. 1997;52(2):149–52.
31. Lavoie KL, Bacon SL, Barone S, Cartier A, Ditto B, Labrecque M. What is worse for asthma control and quality of life: depressive disorders, anxiety disorders, or both? Chest. 2006;130(4):1039–47.
32. Interaction techniques. Motivational interviewing: resources for clinicians, researchers, and trainers; January 2003. http://motivationalinterview.net/clinical/interaction.html
33. Ratanawongsa N, Barton JL, Lyles CR, et al. Association between clinician computer use and communication with patients in safety-net clinics. JAMA Intern Med. 2016;176(1):125–8.
34. Mitchell P, Wynia M, Golden R, et al. Core principles and values of effective team-based health care. National AHEC Organization; October 2012. https://www.nationalahec.org/pdfs/vsrt-team-based-care-principles-values.pdf
35. Hughes LD, Done J, Young A. Not 2 old 2 TXT: there is potential to use email and SMS text message healthcare reminders for rheumatology patients up to 65 years old. Health Informatics J. 2011;17(4):266–76.

36. Sternfeld B, Block C, Quesenberry CP Jr, et al. Improving diet and physical activity with ALIVE: a worksite randomized trial. Am J Prev Med. 2009;36(6):475–83.
37. Montes JM, Medina E, Gomez-Beneyto M, Maurino J. A short message service (SMS)-based strategy for enhancing adherence to antipsychotic medication in schizophrenia. Psychiatry Res. 2012;200(2–3):89–95.
38. Stacy JN, Schwartz SM, Ershoff D, Shreve MS. Incorporating tailored interactive patient solutions using interactive voice response technology to improve statin adherence: results of a randomized clinical trial in a managed care setting. Popul Health Manag. 2009;12(5):241–54.
39. Vollmer WM, Kirshner M, Peters D, et al. Use and impact of an automated telephone outreach system for asthma in a managed care setting. Am J Manag Care. 2006;12(12):725–33.
40. Goldman RE, Sanchez-Hernandez M, Ross-Degnan D, Piette JD, Trinacty CM, Simon SR. Developing an automated speech-recognition telephone diabetes intervention. Int J Qual Health Care. 2008;20(4):264–70.
41. Bender BG, Aloia MS, Rankin AE, Wamboldt FS. Translational behavioral research in respiratory medicine. Chest. 2011;139(6):1279–84.
42. Dimatteo MR. The role of effective communication with children and their families in fostering adherence to pediatric regimens. Patient Educ Couns. 2004;55(3):339–44.
43. Webb SA, Litton E, Barned KL, Crozier TM. Treatment goals: health care improvement through setting and measuring patient-centred outcomes. Crit Care Resusc. 2013;15(2):143–6.
44. Bosworth HB, Olsen MK, Neary A, et al. Take Control of Your Blood Pressure (TCYB) study: a multifactorial tailored behavioral and educational intervention for achieving blood pressure control. Patient Educ Couns. 2008;70(3):338–47.
45. Noble PC, Fuller-Lafreniere S, Meftah M, Dwyer MK. Challenges in outcome measurement: discrepancies between patient and provider definitions of success. Clin Orthop Relat Res. 2013;471(11):3437–45.
46. Bloomrosen M, Sennett C. Patient engagement: challenges and opportunities for physicians. Ann Allergy Asthma Immunol. 2015;115(6):459–62.
47. Coulter A, Stilwell D, Kryworuchko J, Mullen PD, Ng CJ, van der Weijden T. A systematic development process for patient decision aids. BMC Med Inform Decis Mak. 2013;13(Suppl 2):S2.

How Care Coordinators and Other Nursing Professionals Can Help Optimize Care of Asthma in Older Adults

9

Cheryl K. Bernstein and Concettina (Tina) Tolomeo

Introduction

Asthma is a chronic illness. As such, it can have a significant impact on a patient's health and quality of life. Health-related quality of life is an outcome that assesses the impact of a chronic illness on a patient's physical, psychological, emotional, and societal well-being [1]. The impact asthma has on a patient increases with the patient's age [2]. According to the 2015 National Health Interview Survey, current asthma prevalence in people 65 years of age and older in the United States is 6.6%. Furthermore, the prevalence of asthma attacks in this age group is 39.4% [3]. Therefore, a concerted effort must be made to address this vulnerable population. Nurses and care coordinators are in an ideal position to partner with and help make a positive difference in the lives of older adults with asthma. By providing education and care coordination support for older adults with asthma, they can be empowered to practice self-management of their disease and improve their health-related outcomes.

This chapter will provide an overview of asthma education and self-management, care coordination, and the establishment of an effective patient-educator partnership. Additionally, it will introduce adult learner principles as well as provide clinical pearls for the asthma care coordinator.

C. K. Bernstein
Bernstein Clinical Research Center, LLC, Cincinnati, OH, USA
e-mail: cherylkb@bernsteincrc.com

C. Tolomeo (✉)
Yale Medicine and the Department of Pediatrics, Yale School of Medicine,
New Haven, CT, USA
e-mail: tina.tolomeo@yale.edu

© Springer Nature Switzerland AG 2019
T. E. G. Epstein, S. M. Nyenhuis (eds.), *Treatment of Asthma in Older Adults*,
https://doi.org/10.1007/978-3-030-20554-6_9

Asthma Education and Self-Management to Improve Care

Asthma Education

Asthma education is a critical component of asthma management. Studies have shown that asthma education contributes to improved asthma control [4, 5]. Additionally, asthma education has been found to be a cost-effective, nonpharmacologic intervention for asthma management [6]. Although asthma education is advocated, it is not always provided, especially in the older adult population [7]. To complicate matters, older adults often have comorbid conditions leading to polypharmacy. Additionally, they can have visual, memory, and fine motor skills impairments. These factors, coupled with a lack of asthma-specific training, can contribute to poor asthma outcomes in this high-risk population.

It is recommended that asthma education include basic facts about asthma, purpose and use of medications, as well as patient skills training including environmental allergen/trigger avoidance strategies, self-monitoring techniques, and use of an asthma action plan [4]. While necessary, these components of asthma education can be overwhelming and difficult for some patients to grasp. Therefore, they should be introduced in a stepwise fashion. Furthermore, when planning an asthma education program for older adults, it is important to consider the factors (comorbidities, polypharmacy, and impairments) noted above. Such factors may have implications for the plan of care. For instance, a patient with decreased dexterity may have difficulty using a metered dose inhaler and may have more success with a breath-actuated device if he or she is able to generate an appropriate inspiratory flow rate.

As important as the education itself, it is imperative that the training include an assessment of the concepts presented. This can be done by asking the patient open-ended questions such as "Where will you keep your asthma action plan?", "Which medication would you use if you were wheezing?", and "What would you do if your wheezing did not respond to albuterol?". In addition to asthma-specific education, patients need support and guidance to help them effectively manage their disease.

Asthma Self-Management

Self-management is the process by which the patient actively assumes day-to-day management of his or her chronic illness [8, 9]. Because asthma is a chronic disease, the need to practice self-management is lifelong. There are three self-management tasks the patient must master: (1) medical management (i.e., taking medication), (2) role management (i.e., avoiding cigarette smoke), and (3) emotional management (i.e., coping with the fear of steroids). Additionally, required self-management skills include problem-solving, decision-making, resource utilization, development of a patient-provider partnership, action planning, and applying self-management skills to oneself [8]. Self-management has been utilized in several chronic illnesses including asthma, diabetes, and arthritis, to name a few. Studies of asthma self-management have varied in content, duration, and resources, thereby making it difficult to determine which techniques are most effective. Self-management techniques that have been studied and implemented include group classes, one-on-one education, provision of written materials, electronic/web-based programs, telephone support/training, and combinations thereof. Despite the variety, one thing holds true: self-management has been found to improve healthcare outcomes [10–12].

To be effective, self-management should be personalized to meet the patient's needs. Baptist et al. [10] conducted a study to determine common asthma self-management challenges encountered by older adults. Findings revealed that the following were viewed as challenges for the older adults studied: (1) atypical asthma symptoms, (2) inability to distinguish asthma from other medical conditions, (3) asthma medication concerns and compliance, (4) use of complementary and alternative therapies, (5) a desire for independence in asthma management, and (6) the need for asthma education programs for older adults. In another study, Miles et al. [11] conducted a review of qualitative research regarding asthma self-management to determine the barriers and facilitators associated with effective asthma self-management strategies. Eleven barrier/facilitator themes emerged from this review, some of which overlapped with the study conducted by Baptist et al. [10]. The themes were (1) partnership between patient and healthcare professional, (2) issues around medication, (3) education about asthma and its management, (4) health beliefs, (5) self-management interventions, (6) comorbidities, (7) mood disorders and anxiety, (8) social support, (9) nonpharmacological methods, (10) access to healthcare, and (11) professional factors in the healthcare system such as insufficient time during a visit and lack of communication among providers.

To maximize the positive effects of self-management, barriers must be addressed and overcome. Suggestions for minimizing barriers include [4, 10, 11]:

- Maintain open lines of communication with the patient without being judgmental.
- Elicit patient goals and beliefs so they can be incorporated into the plan of care.
- Make every interaction a teachable moment.
- Review with the patient his/her own asthma signs and symptoms.
- Provide information that is concise and culturally appropriate using layperson terms.
- Provide language and culturally appropriate written materials at the 5th grade reading level.
- Review the patient's medication list to avoid interactions and side effects.
- Identify barriers to obtaining medications and intervene as necessary (i.e., provide medication samples, enroll in free/reduced care programs, etc.).
- Provide and review a mutually agreed-upon asthma action plan.
- Institute strategies to help the patient remember to take medications (i.e., medication/pill boxes, alarms, automatic pharmacy refills/delivery service, etc.).
- Encourage the patient to enlist the help (including attending appointments and providing medication reminders) of friends and family members.

- Utilize community resources (i.e., visiting nurses, support groups, medical rides, etc.).
- Provide coordination of care services to help patients navigate appointments, medication prior authorizations, etc.
- Expand your knowledge of asthma care and self-management.

Asthma Educators as Care Coordinators

Care Coordination

Coordination of patient care has become a top priority for healthcare decision-makers, given the current emphasis on quality, patient-centered care, the aging population, and our increasingly complex healthcare systems [13, 14]. Care coordination has been defined numerous ways. One broad definition of care coordination is "the deliberate organization of patient care activities between two or more participants (including the patient) involved in a patient's care to facilitate the appropriate delivery of health care services" [13, 14]. This involves uniting and communicating with others participating in the patient's care and securing the necessary resources to ensure optimal care is met. The overall goals of care coordination are to organize the patients care services and improve health outcomes. Related terms include case or care management, disease management, and patient navigation. Case or care management involves assigning the responsibility for guiding a patient through the care process in an effective and efficient manner to a case or care manager or team. Disease management refers to the coordination and integration of healthcare services in order to manage a patient's chronic disease. It emphasizes the concepts of education and self-management. Patient navigation entails helping patients steer their way through the complex health system in order to access quality care. A common theme among all terms is helping patients access appropriate care in an efficient manner [12–14].

Effective care coordinators have knowledge of both the patient and the healthcare system. Additionally, they are adept at engaging the patient and navigating the healthcare system [15]. To engage patients in managing their care, care coordinators must be proficient in coaching and teaching. These are concepts with which asthma educators are very familiar.

Asthma Educators

Asthma educators can play a key role in helping older adults manage their asthma. Asthma educators have been defined as "experts in teaching, educating, and counseling individuals with asthma and their families in the knowledge and skills necessary to minimize the impact of asthma on their quality of life" [16]. As such, they are well suited to serve as care coordinators. Asthma educators come from a variety of disciplines including, but not limited to, nursing, social work, and respiratory therapy. They make significant contributions in the hospital, ambulatory, and homecare settings. Asthma educators provide education about the disease process; coordination of care services (with other healthcare providers, insurance carriers, etc.); information and connection to appropriate community resources; as well as support and advice to patients who have questions or need clarification regarding their plan of care.

National certification for asthma educators became available in the United States in September of 2002. The certifying body is the National Asthma Educator Certification Board (NAECB). The NAECB ensures those who have successfully achieved certification have a well-founded understanding of the scientific concepts required to perform the functions of an asthma educator. To be eligible for the examination, the educator must be a licensed practical nurse, nurse practitioner, registered nurse, physician, physician assistant, respiratory therapist, pulmonary function technologist, pharmacist, social worker, health educator, occupational therapist, physical therapist, or an individual who has provided asthma education or coordination of services with a minimum of 1000 hours worked. The asthma certification designation is AE-C. The certification exam consists of 175 questions. Exam categories include the asthma condition, patient and family assessment, asthma management, and organizational issues. Recertification is available by testing or by continuing education credits [16].

Partnership in Care

Strong Patient/Nurse Partnership

Establishing a strong working relationship between the patient and the nurse is essential for developing mutual respect, a safe and secure environment, and trust. Working together building a strong patient/nurse partnership will allow the patient to feel part of the "team" and decision-making process. This open exchange of information and communication should help reveal the patient's true goals and objectives.

Mutual Goals of Asthma Management

Recognizing and identifying the patient's asthma goals and objectives are key to developing an asthma treatment guide and management plan. It is helpful to start by asking the patient, "What would you like to be able to do that you are unable to do because of your asthma?" Then listen carefully, and the patient might reply, "I want to be able to play with my grandchild, go to the park, do laundry, play golf, shop, walk up a flight of steps, get a good night sleep, etc." The lifestyle goals are endless, but specific to that individual. Maybe the older adult patient has arthritis and does not have fine motor control, which would affect their ability to take certain asthma inhalers and medications or is unable to hear or see well. Some patients may have difficulty understanding simple directions, while others are well connected to social media and computers. Establishing a framework regarding their unique goals and objectives are key to designing an effective and relevant treatment education program. Regardless of the patient's abilities, it is very helpful to have family members present during this process. Family members, significant others, and close friends can hear and participate in the communication process, and help the patient remember events that affected their quality of life. Such contacts might help recall specific asthma symptoms or medical events that were limiting, or even scary to the patient. They might add additional goals and objectives based on realistic lifetime challenges.

Establishing this type of open communication will assist the healthcare professional to speak directly to the patient's specific goals and incorporate them into explaining how, when, and why to take their asthma medications. If the patient understands how the medications work and how they will directly impact their activities, they might be more motivated to be compliant with their treatment. "Connecting the dots" between the asthma medication and the patient's activities, goals, and objectives help to bring the concepts to a more concrete and realistic level for the patient. The patient sometimes does not completely understand that their feeling of "wellness" and asthma control are directly linked to taking their medication regime as prescribed.

A Case Study

A 68-year-old African-American female with a confirmed history of physician diagnosed asthma came into the office complaining of increased nighttime awakenings, increased albuterol usage during the day and night, shortness of breath during slight exertion, and wheezing. The patient admitted that she stopped taking her asthma controller medication since her asthma seemed well controlled and that she did not believe she needed the treatment any longer. She verbalized that the medication was very expensive and was not worth the money and was not much help. She thought that her asthma was cured. Her spirometry revealed that she had a 20% drop in FEV-1 since her last visit 6 months ago. She denied symptoms of fever, chills, runny nose, cough, and sinus congestion. She verbalized that she was not sure why she was having trouble and complained that she is not able to play with or babysit her grandson who is 2 years old.

The patient was diagnosed with an asthma exacerbation and was prescribed oral corticosteroids and an asthma controller medication. The patient verbalized that she was completely surprised that her worsening asthma was due to stopping her controller asthma therapy. She explained that she was afraid that she would become addicted to the medication and therefore decided to stop taking it daily since she felt so well.

The patient was reassured during the visit and encouraged to ask many questions regarding her asthma and medication treatment plan. She demonstrated her inhaler technique, which provided an excellent opportunity to re-educate and correct her dosing methods. A new asthma action plan was designed specifically for the patient and tailored to the patient's life style. Her concerns regarding addiction to the treatment were carefully addressed, and a frequent follow-up plan was scheduled with the prescribing provider. The patient was encouraged to call for any questions or problems. The patient agreed to call before changing or stopping the prescribed treatment plan.

Communicating Effectively

Communicating and carefully listening to the patients' questions and answers provides valuable insights into the likelihood that the patients will be compliant with the treatment. For example, the patient may ask the following: "What if I forget to take my morning or evening asthma medication?"; "Is it really necessary to take the medication twice a day?"; "Why do I need to take so many puffs a day, it seems to use up the medication quickly"; "I sometimes have trouble remembering my medication even if I check it off on my calendar"; or "The inhalers are expensive and I am not sure if they will be covered by insurance." These questions reveal that the patient has doubt regarding their ability to remain compliant with the treatment and adhere to the plan. Problem-solving for the patient is essential and might involve reviewing the patient's pharmacy formulary and discussing the treatment plan with the provider. The full team including the patient should be included in the decision-making process. Finding the best, most affordable and effective asthma treatment plan that the patient understands and agrees to follow will help ensure compliance and adherence. Each visit the provider and nurse should review the plan with the patient and assess understanding and compliance. It is important to emphasize taking the medication as agreed and calling the office to discuss alternative plans before stopping or changing the treatment plan. The patient's perceptions of the medication and treatment plan and willingness to follow the directions are all crucial to the overall success and effectiveness of the communication.

Problem-Solving Misperceptions

According to Marcey Aronson, one of the authors and program developers of "Learn Brainzones," adult learners need to have an open mind to accept information, especially if they already are following and implementing a contrary way of thinking [17]. Talking to the patient in a calm and relaxed voice creates a calm trusting environment that is needed to change the attitudes of negative thinking. Identifying and discussing the patient's goals and presenting solutions will help lead the adult learner to anticipate consequences. For example, if the patient's goal is to actively participate in daily activities with his/her family and friends, it is important that they comprehend the consequences of failure to follow their asthma action plan. The ability to develop insight regarding their asthma control level is crucial and key for proper decision-making and acceptance of their personalized treatment plan. The patient's feelings and emotional involvement regarding living with a chronic illness

Table 9.1 Key patient educational concepts

Incorporate the patient's information to personalize the educational session

Organize the presentation with the most important and relevant information first followed by the least

Set priorities and reinforce the information, by repeating it several times to the patient

Allow time for questions and provide praise to the patient frequently

Speak slowly keeping the information simple and avoid using medical terminology and complicated vocabulary

Use simple numbers during the discussion and avoid using percentages, especially if the patient has an indication of impaired health literacy

Use analogies when possible and ask the patient to discuss the information

Avoid asking if they understand, but rather use open-ended sentences and communication to facilitate open dialogue and information exchange

Use illustrations, drawings, pictures, tables, and graphs to emphasize the main points

Watch for nonverbal communication such as poor eye contact and yawning

Encourage active participation and redirect if the patient or family members appear to be disinterested in the session

Frequently offer praise and reassurance during the educational session and continue to encourage questions and open communication

can affect their ability to listen and accept the information. Finding ways to effectively connect with the adult learner with positive, respectful, and open communication will maximize their feeling of collaboration and enhance leaning (Table 9.1).

Adult Learners

Literacy

It is important to determine the educational level and literacy of the adult learner prior to starting the asthma education process. Health literacy is defined according to The Global Initiative for Asthma as the "degree to which individuals have the capacity to obtain, process and understand basic health information and services to make appropriate health decisions" [5]. If a patient has low health literacy, with decreased knowledge and understanding, education is difficult and can result in poor asthma control and outcomes. The nurse must find other methods of communication that reduce the negative impact of poor health literacy. The partnership is essential to overcoming the overwhelming barriers. Establishing communication strategies tailored to meet the needs of each individual patient is essential for effective patient education. This includes adjusting to cultural differences, misconceptions, and beliefs that impact health literacy.

Learning Methods/Techniques

The case coordinator/nurse professional needs to be friendly, knowledgeable, and show interest and sincere concern for the patient. Many patients, and particularly older adults, enjoy speaking about their families, hobbies, and interests, and should be encouraged to share their experiences. Open communication will allow the patient to verbalize their goals, beliefs, concerns, and value systems. What are they hoping to achieve because of their treatment? Do they want to be able to do daily activities and exercise and keep up with grandchildren, family members, and pets?

Asthma-Specific Education

The nurse should demonstrate the proper inhaler technique using trainers. The patient should also use the inhaler trainers however, when appropriate, use their own asthma medication. Confirm patient and family asthma knowledge by providing return demonstration opportunities at each office visit. The patient should physically demonstrate the proper technique for using asthma inhalers. If the patient verbalizes or demonstrates that they are having difficulty mastering the proper inhaler technique, or are not able to properly take the prescribed medication, the provider/physician needs to be informed. Additional education can be repeated, but new prescribed medication might be indicated based on the patient's cognitive level, physical abilities, and limitations. Patient education and re-education are crucial to ensure adherence at each office visit and patient encounter. Provide praise and re-educate as needed.

Clinical Pearls for the Asthma Care Coordinator

- Provide patients, significant others, and family members with your office contact information and encourage them to add the contact to their phone so that they always have your number readily available. If appropriate, provide mobile phone numbers and email for direct and easy access.
- Be cognizant of common problems with asthma self-management and provide anticipatory guidance:
  - Inappropriately discontinuing controller medications when symptoms resolve and overuse of quick-relief medications. It is important to explain what each type of medication does in terms the patient can understand. Determine if the patient accepts the information and if they agree to take as directed. If the patient continues to verbalize doubt and confusion regarding the treatment plan, continue to educate and if needed schedule support follow-up education.
  - Incorrect use and cleaning of inhalation therapy devices. It is important to assess inhaler technique at each visit. This can be done with the use of an objective device called the In-Check Dial (http://www.alliancetechmedical.com/products/check-dial-training-device/).
  - Misplacing asthma action plan. Help the patient decide on a prominent location for the action plan.
- To aid the patient's understanding of inflammation, utilize diagrams and airway models when providing asthma education.

- Use simple vocabulary and avoid medical terminology.
- Don't assume the patient understood the information provided. Use open-ended questions and ask him/her to repeat their understanding of the material using their own words.
- Ask the patient if they agree with their asthma action plan, and if they feel their goals and objectives have been met. If the patient verbalizes doubt or concern, reassess and modify the plan.
- Include the patient's significant other, family members, or close friends during asthma education and medication instructions to provide support and reinforce the asthma self-care management to the patient.
- Encourage the patient to contact you if they have problems obtaining medications or if they have concerns.

Conclusion

Asthma education and self-management are essential components of asthma care and management. Care coordination contributes to the successful management of chronic illnesses such as asthma. Asthma educators are well prepared to function in the care coordinator role. In this role, asthma care coordinators have the knowledge and expertise necessary to positively impact the lives of older adults with asthma. Nurses and other healthcare professionals who are not certified asthma educators can also impact the lives of the older adult patient by incorporating adult learning principles and encouraging partnered decision-making and self-management.

References

1. Urbstonaitis R, Deshpande M, Arnoldi J. Asthma and health related quality of life in late midlife adults. Res Soc Adm Pharm. 2018; https://doi.org/10.1016/j.sapharm.2018.03.003.
2. Goeman D, Jenkins C, Crane M, Paul E, Douglass J. Educational intervention for older people with asthma: a randomized controlled trial. Patient Educ Couns. 2013;93:586–95.
3. Centers for Disease Control and Prevention (CDC). 2015 National health interview survey; 2015. https://www.cdc.gov/asthma/nhis/2015/data.htm. Accessed 30 Mar 2018.
4. National Heart Lung and Blood Institute (NHLBI), National Asthma Education and Prevention Program (NAEPP). Expert panel report 3: guidelines for the diagnosis and management of asthma. US Department of Health and Human Services; 2007. https://www.nhlbi.nih.gov/sites/default/files/media/docs/asthgdln_1.pdf. Accessed 30 Mar 2018.
5. Global Initiative for Asthma (GINA). Global strategy for asthma management and prevention; 2018. https://ginasthma.org/wp-content/uploads/2018/04/wms-GINA-2018-report-V1.3-002.pdf. Accessed 3 Mar 2019.
6. Crossman-Barnes CJ, Peel A, Fng-Soe-Khioe R, Sach T, Wilson A, Barton G. Economic evidence for nonpharmacological asthma management interventions: a systematic review. Allergy. 2017; https://doi.org/10.1111/all.13337.
7. Ozturk AB, Ozyigit Pur L, Kostek O, Keskin H. Association between asthma self-management knowledge and asthma control in the elderly. Ann Allergy Asthma Immunol. 2015;114:480–4.
8. Lorig KR, Holman HR. Self-management education: history, definition, outcomes, and mechanisms. Ann Behav Med. 2003;26:1–7.

9. Schulman-Green D, Jaser S, Martin F, Alonzo A, Grey M, McCorkle R, et al. Processes of self-management in chronic illness. J Nurs Scholarsh. 2012;44:136–44. https://doi.org/10.1111/j.1547-5069.2012.01444.x.

10. Baptist AP, Deol BBK, Reddy RR, Nelson B, Clark NM. Age-specific factors influencing asthma management by older adults. Qual Health Res. 2010;20:117–24. https://doi.org/10.1177/1049732309355288.

11. Miles C, Arden-Close E, Thomas M, Bruton A, Yardley L, Hankins M, et al. Barriers and facilitators of effective self-management in asthma: systematic review and thematic synthesis of patient and healthcare professional views. Prim Care Respir Med. 2017:27–57. https://doi.org/10.1038/s41533-017-0056-4.

12. Peytremann-Bridevaux I, Arditi C, Gex G, Bridevaux PO, Burnand B. Chronic disease management programmes for adults with asthma. Cochrane Database Syst Rev. 2015;(5):CD007988. https://doi.org/10.1002/14651858.CD007988.pub2.

13. Shojania KG, McDonald KM, Wachter RM, Owens DK. Care coordination. In: Closing the quality gap: a critical analysis of quality improvement strategies. Agency for Healthcare Research and Quality Publication No. 04(07)-0051-7; 2007. https://www.ahrq.gov/downloads/pub/evidence/pdf/caregap/caregap.pdf Accessed 30 Mar 2018.

14. Schultz EM, McDonald KM. What is care coordination? Int J Care Coord. 2014;17:5–24. https://doi.org/10.1177/2053435414540615.

15. Izumi S, Barfield PA, Basin B, Mood L, Neunzert C, Tadesse R, et al. Care coordination: identifying and connecting the most appropriate care to the patients. Res Nurs Health. 2018;41:49–56. https://doi.org/10.1002/nur.21843.

16. National Asthma Educator Certification Board (NAECB). Certified asthma educator AE-C: candidate handbook; 2018. https://naecb.com/certificants/get-certified/exam-information/. Accessed 3 Mar 2019.

17. Aronson M, Leonard D. "Learn Brainzones" social, emotional program designed to understand, recognize and self-regulate your emotions. Brainzones, LLC: Akron; 2018.

Asthma Phenotypes of Older Adults

10

Sameer K. Mathur

Introduction

It is well recognized that asthma is a heterogeneous disease. There are many initiatives to categorize subtypes or phenotypes of asthma with respect to composition of airway inflammatory cells, clinical features, or predominant molecular signals/pathways. These efforts have successfully identified many phenotypes of asthma; however, the clinical relevance of these remains to be fully realized. It is expected that identifying asthma phenotypes will lead to optimized management strategies for each respective phenotype. For older patients with asthma, there is an additional layer of complexity regarding phenotypes. Specifically, does an older asthma patient have the same phenotype of asthma as they did when younger? If so, does the older age version of the phenotype have clinically relevant age-related differences? Alternatively, do younger patients transition into one of a new set of older asthma phenotypes depending on exposures, infections, obesity, and disease activity? Unfortunately, these are questions that are yet to be answered. This chapter will discuss efforts to phenotype asthma and our understanding of implications for asthma in older adults. It is clear that we are at only the beginning stages of realizing the goal of defining clinically relevant asthma phenotypes along the entire age spectrum.

Methods of Phenotyping Asthma

The earliest efforts to phenotype asthma were based on simplistic clinical descriptors associated with the asthma symptoms such as exercise-induced, virus-induced, extrinsic, or intrinsic. A more comprehensive method of

S. K. Mathur (✉)
Department of Medicine, University of Wisconsin School of Medicine and Public Health, Madison, WI, USA
e-mail: skmathur@wisc.edu

© Springer Nature Switzerland AG 2019
T. E. G. Epstein, S. M. Nyenhuis (eds.), *Treatment of Asthma in Older Adults*, https://doi.org/10.1007/978-3-030-20554-6_10

phenotyping involved considering additional clinical features (e.g., severity, exacerbation-prone, treatment-resistant), triggers of disease activity (e.g., allergic-driven, aspirin-induced, occupational), and composition of airway inflammation (e.g., neutrophilic, eosinophilic, paucigranulocytic) [1]. However, these combined clinical features and airway characteristics have a great deal of overlap, such that distinct clinically meaningful subsets of asthma were not easily discerned.

More sophisticated statistical approaches, often referred to as "hierarchical cluster analysis" or "latent class analysis," have led to more recent efforts to phenotype patients. These approaches essentially allow patient data to "sort themselves" within some defined constraints into clusters or phenotypes of disease.

Phenotypes of Severe Asthma

The United States based, NIH-sponsored, Severe Asthma Research Program (SARP) first published results using hierarchical cluster analysis from a cross-sectional analysis of 726 patients to define 5 clusters of patients using 34 clinical variables [2]. Notably, one of the clusters had a predominance of "late-onset asthma" patients. Furthermore, another cluster included predominantly older patients with low baseline and postbronchodilator forced expiratory volume in 1 second (FEV1). Since age was included as a clinical variable for the analysis, it is not clear whether younger and older asthma patients would independently distribute into the same or different clusters. Nevertheless, there was a clear indication that some clinical characteristics did track along with older age.

It is expected that the inclusion of biological variables in the cluster analysis will provide additional details for the phenotypes to better define mechanisms of disease, and this type of clustering is referred to as "endotypes". In the reanalysis of a subset of 378 patients from the SARP cohort including biological variables from the bronchoscopy, peripheral blood, and the fractionated exhaled nitric oxide (FeNO) for a total of 112 variables, six clusters were identified [3]. Two of the clusters had patients older than the other clusters, one of which included mostly patients with late-onset asthma. The other older cluster had childhood-onset asthma, but both of the clusters had more severe disease as noted by increased physician office visits, increased emergency room visits, and increased intensive-care unit admissions.

In a cluster analysis of another subset of 155 patients from the SARP cohort, the gene-expression profile from bronchial epithelial cells was used for cluster analysis without inclusion of clinical variables [4]. The genes used for the cluster analysis were those that exhibited a significant correlation (positive or negative) with the FeNO levels. This analysis identified five clusters; however, no one cluster consisted of a greater proportion of the older subjects. Interestingly, there was one cluster that had mostly younger patients, with older subjects spread among the other four clusters. This raises the possibility that biological mechanisms involved in asthma may be age-independent.

Phenotypes of Older Asthma

In a Korean study, cluster analysis was performed using nine clinical variables in asthma patients over 65 years of age with data from two separate cohorts, one to generate the clusters (872 patients) and the second for validation (429 patients) [5]. Their analysis identified four clusters, one characterized by long symptom duration and one of which had mostly smokers, which likely represents a group with the asthma COPD overlap syndrome. The cluster with smokers and another cluster were notable for high proportion of atopic patients. In addition, it was noted that one of the nonatopic clusters represented more severe disease with a shorter time to first exacerbation compared to the other clusters.

In a recent cluster analysis of 180 older asthma patients (all above 55 years of age), four clusters were identified [6]. One cluster had a later onset of asthma with corresponding less duration of asthma. The second cluster had mild asthma. The third cluster had early onset of asthma and highest prevalence of atopy. The fourth cluster had the most severe disease, as suggested by the lowest asthma control test scores and lowest prebronchodilator FEV1.

Although the use of cluster analyses provides guidance for phenotypes of asthma for research purposes, the broad based clinical utility of these phenotypes can only be realized if the determination of phenotype can be performed with only a few easily obtained variables. For example, the initial cluster designations of the SARP cohort could be fairly reliably assigned by examining only three variables: baseline FEV1, maximum postbronchodilator FEV1, and age of asthma onset [2]. It is likely that other biomarkers may also serve such a role in a limited subset of variables for assignment of phenotype. However, in older adults, this must be done cautiously as biomarkers may have different characteristics in younger and older asthma patients. For example, the identification of sputum neutrophilia as a marker for more severe asthma [7] has also been observed to be a characteristic feature of older asthma patients with mild disease [8].

Stability of Asthma Phenotypes Over Time

In order to address whether asthma phenotypes are stable, data from three European long-term follow-up asthma cohort studies were combined, the European Community Respiratory Health Survey (ECRHS), the Epidemiological Study on Genetics and Environment of Asthma (EGEA), and the Swiss Cohort Study on Air Pollution and Lung and Heart Disease in Adults (SAPALDIA) [9]. Analysis of this combined cohort of 3320 patients identified seven baseline clusters based on nine clinical variables. Two of the clusters had greater proportions of older patients (i.e., greater odds of age >40 at baseline) compared to the other clusters, specifically one nonallergic with high symptoms and the other allergic with moderate symptoms and presence of bronchial hyperreactivity. The older cluster with high symptoms was also notable for having the highest odds of reporting subsequent asthma exacerbation in one year. In comparing the cluster designations of individual patients from their baseline to the follow-up visit approximately 10 years later, it was observed that there was variation in how many patients stayed within their initial cluster designation (54–88%). With respect to the two clusters with older patients, the nonallergic, high symptom cluster had 73% of patients remain in the same cluster with the majority (15%) of others transitioning into the nonallergic, few symptom cluster. The allergic, moderate symptoms cluster had 88% of patients remain in the same cluster, with the majority (11%) of others transitioning to allergic with high symptoms. Thus, the nonallergic older patients stayed the same or improved, while the allergic older patients stayed the same or worsened.

In a longitudinal study of 171 adult-onset asthma patients (diagnosed at age 15 years or older), five baseline clusters were identified, two of which included smokers [10]. Of the other three, one cluster was 98% female with normal lung function and moderate levels of both symptoms and health-care utilizations. Another cluster was notable for obesity, uncontrolled asthma symptoms despite medication use, greatest level of comorbidities, and highest healthcare utilization. The final cluster had younger patients, was more atopic, and had greatest bronchodilator reversibility on lung function. In this study, cluster analysis was not performed again at the 12-year follow-up; rather, the focus was to establish the long-term outcomes from the initial cluster designation. Interestingly, one of the notable changes over the 12-year observation period was a decline in blood eosinophil count in all the clusters except one of the smoking clusters.

Asthma-COPD Overlap Syndrome

There has been recent interest and acknowledgment that a significant number of older patients may have the asthma-COPD overlap syndrome (ACOS) [11]. In a recent study of 161 asthma and COPD patients, it was demonstrated that cluster analysis using clinical features biological readouts from the sputum, clusters can be defined to differentiate the three diagnoses of asthma, COPD, and ACOS [12]. This serves as a reminder that comorbidities, which are more commonly seen in older adults, can impact both clinical and biological variables.

Utility of Asthma Phenotype for Disease Management

Omalizumab (Xolair) can be considered the first phenotype specific asthma therapy approved by the Food and Drug Administration (FDA) in 2003. This is a humanized anti-IgE antibody that is approved for use in an allergic severe asthma phenotype. However, it is known that total IgE levels and allergic sensitization decline with age [13, 14]; thus, there was concern as to whether omalizumab would be effective in older asthma patients. In a study comparing response to omalizumab in patients above and below age 50 years, reductions in rates of exacerbations were comparable: 68.9% in patients equal or above age 50 years and 75.4% in patients below age 50 years [15]. There have also been FDA approvals of three medications for use in another asthma phenotype of severe eosinophilic asthma: mepolizumab (Nucala) in 2015, reslizumab (Cinqair) in 2016, and benralizumab (Fasenra) in 2017 [16]. These have all been used in a variety of age groups, with the most recent pivotal studies for mepolizumab enrolling up to age 82 [17], reslizumab up to age 75 [18], and benralizumab up to age 75 [19, 20]. Finally, dupilumab (Dupixent) was approved in 2018 for moderate-to-severe eosinophilic asthma or corticosteroid-dependent asthma, with the pivotal studies enrolling patients with mean ages of 49–51 with standard deviation of 12–15 years [21, 22]. However, whether there is a differential efficacy in older asthma patients versus younger has not been specifically addressed.

Summary

There is a great deal of interest and promise in the efforts to identify phenotypes of asthma. The work thus far with cross-sectional studies has demonstrated that phenotypes can be established based on clinical assessments, biological assessments, and their combination. There is a great need to include older asthma patients in studies identifying phenotypes and endotypes, i.e., above age 65 years old. Furthermore, more longitudinal studies are also needed to better assess the stability and potential transitions of phenotypes over time. Ultimately, the hope is to be able to intervene on specific asthma phenotypes at early ages to influence a transition into "older age" phenotypes of asthma that are better controlled and have minimal healthcare utilization.

References

1. Wenzel SE. Asthma: defining of the persistent adult phenotypes. Lancet. 2006;368:804–13.
2. Moore WC, Meyers DA, Wenzel SE, et al. Identification of asthma phenotypes using cluster analysis in the Severe Asthma Research Program. Am J Respir Crit Care Med. 2010;181:315–23.
3. Wu W, Bleecker E, Moore W, et al. Unsupervised phenotyping of Severe Asthma Research Program participants using expanded lung data. J Allergy Clin Immunol. 2014;133:1280–8.
4. Modena BD, Tedrow JR, Milosevic J, et al. Gene expression in relation to exhaled nitric oxide identifies novel asthma phenotypes with unique biomolecular pathways. Am J Respir Crit Care Med. 2014;190:1363–72.
5. Park HW, Song WJ, Kim SH, et al. Classification and implementation of asthma phenotypes in elderly patients. Annals of allergy, asthma & immunology: official publication of the American College of Allergy, Asthma. Immunology. 2015;114:18–22.
6. Baptist AP, Hao W, Karamched KR, et al. Distinct asthma phenotypes among older adults with asthma. J Allergy Clin Immunol Pract. 2018;6:244–249.e242.
7. Jatakanon A, Uasuf C, Maziak W, et al. Neutrophilic inflammation in severe persistent asthma. Am J Respir Crit Care Med. 1999;160:1532–9.
8. Nyenhuis SM, Schwantes EA, Evans MD, et al. Airway neutrophil inflammatory phenotype in older subjects with asthma. J Allergy Clin Immunol. 2010;125:1163–5.
9. Boudier A, Curjuric I, Basagana X, et al. Ten-year follow-up of cluster-based asthma phenotypes in adults. A pooled analysis of three cohorts. Am J Respir Crit Care Med. 2013;188:550–60.
10. Ilmarinen P, Tuomisto LE, Niemela O, et al. Cluster analysis on longitudinal data of patients with adult-onset asthma. J Allergy Clin Immunol Pract. 2017;5:967–78.e963.

11. Postma DS, Rabe KF. The asthma-COPD overlap syndrome. N Engl J Med. 2015;373:1241–9.
12. Ghebre MA, Bafadhel M, Desai D, et al. Biological clustering supports both "Dutch" and "British" hypotheses of asthma and chronic obstructive pulmonary disease. J Allergy Clin Immunol. 2015;135:63–72.
13. Gergen PJ, Turkeltaub PC, Sempos CT. Is allergen skin test reactivity a predictor of mortality? Findings from a national cohort. Clin Exp Allergy. 2000;30:1717–23.
14. Barbee RA, Halonen M, Lebowitz M, et al. Distribution of Ige in a community population-sample – correlations with age, sex, and allergen skin-test reactivity. J Allergy Clin Immunol. 1981;68:106–11.
15. Korn S, Schumann C, Kropf C, et al. Effectiveness of omalizumab in patients 50 years and older with severe persistent allergic asthma. Ann Allergy Asthma Immunol. 2010;105:313–9.
16. Manka LA, Wechsler ME. Selecting the right biologic for your patients with severe asthma. Annals of allergy, asthma & immunology: official publication of the American College of Allergy, Asthma. Immunology. 2018;121:406–13.
17. Ortega HG, Liu MC, Pavord ID, et al. Mepolizumab treatment in patients with severe eosinophilic asthma. N Engl J Med. 2014;371:1198–207.
18. Castro M, Zangrilli J, Wechsler ME, et al. Reslizumab for inadequately controlled asthma with elevated blood eosinophil counts: results from two multicentre, parallel, double-blind, randomised, placebo-controlled, phase 3 trials. Lancet Respir Med. 2015;3:355–66.
19. Bleecker ER, FitzGerald JM, Chanez P, et al. Efficacy and safety of benralizumab for patients with severe asthma uncontrolled with high-dosage inhaled corticosteroids and long-acting beta2-agonists (SIROCCO): a randomised, multicentre, placebo-controlled phase 3 trial. Lancet. 2016;388:2115–27.
20. FitzGerald JM, Bleecker ER, Nair P, et al. Benralizumab, an anti-interleukin-5 receptor alpha monoclonal antibody, as add-on treatment for patients with severe, uncontrolled, eosinophilic asthma (CALIMA): a randomised, double-blind, placebo-controlled phase 3 trial. Lancet. 2016;388:2128–41.
21. Castro M, Corren J, Pavord ID, et al. Dupilumab efficacy and safety in moderate-to-severe uncontrolled asthma. N Engl J Med. 2018;378:2486–96.
22. Rabe KF, Nair P, Brusselle G, et al. Efficacy and safety of dupilumab in glucocorticoid-dependent severe asthma. N Engl J Med. 2018;378:2475–85.

Controlling Triggers for Asthma in Older Adults: Environmental Allergens, Indoor and Outdoor Air Pollutants, and Infection

11

Marissa R. Shams and Tolly E. G. Epstein

As discussed in earlier chapters, asthma impacts between 4.5% and 13% of adults over age 65 years [1]. Asthma in older adults can generally be categorized into two groups: patients with a long-standing history of asthma and those with onset of symptoms after age 65 years [2, 3]. Regardless of the timing of onset, asthmatic patients greater than age 65 have greater morbidity and mortality in comparison to their younger counterparts. As with younger populations, asthma exacerbations and poor asthma control in older adults are often due to a variety of allergic and non-allergic triggers, including indoor allergens, respiratory infections, and pollution (indoor and outdoor). For reasons that will be discussed below, older adults may be more susceptible to the impact of these triggers [1, 4]. An environmental history is therefore key to identifying potential triggers and targets for remediation and prevention in this population.

Aeroallergens

Although atopy is less common in asthmatics over age 65 years than in younger asthmatics, it still impacts a significant number of older adults [2]. It is unclear if immune senescence may impact specific aeroallergen sensitivity and reactivity; however, the association between allergy and asthma clearly persists in a subset of

M. R. Shams (✉)
Division of Pulmonary, Allergy, Critical Care and Sleep Medicine, Department of Internal Medicine, Emory University Hospital, Emory University School of Medicine, Atlanta, GA, USA
e-mail: marissa.reiter.shams@emory.edu

T. E. G. Epstein
Division of Immunology, Allergy, and Rheumatology, University of Cincinnati School of Medicine, Cincinnati, OH, USA
e-mail: epsteite@uc.edu

© Springer Nature Switzerland AG 2019
T. E. G. Epstein, S. M. Nyenhuis (eds.), *Treatment of Asthma in Older Adults*,
https://doi.org/10.1007/978-3-030-20554-6_11

the older adult population [1, 2]. In a recent study involving 243 older adults with asthma in Brazil, allergic asthma was observed in 62.9% of the cohort. A higher prevalence of atopy was identified in those with asthma symptom onset at age less than 12 years (72.1%), and decreased gradually with increased age of asthma-symptom onset [2]. The same study identified the most frequent inhalant sensitizations in this age group as house dust mites, furry pets, and cockroach in 91.5%, 24.8%, and 21.6% of their cohort, respectively [2]. Rogers et al. similarly reported that in a New York City specialty asthma clinic, approximately 60% of asthmatics over age 65 were sensitized to at least one allergen, although the most common sensitization was to cockroach allergen [5]. Yet another study conducted in New York City determined that 41% of adults greater than age 60 with moderate-severe persistent asthma were sensitized to at least one allergen [6]. These values reveal a high rate of allergic sensitization in the elderly, although lower than that of young asthmatic children, in whom 80% are atopic [1]. Epidemiological studies have revealed that asthmatics of any age sensitized to indoor allergens tend to have more severe disease. Sensitization to an indoor inhalant allergen is a risk factor for asthma development [1, 7]. As modern life has shifted toward more time indoors, the association between indoor allergens and asthma severity has become even more relevant [7].

Given the persistence of aeroallergen sensitization, aeroallergen avoidance strategies and environmental control measures play an important role in managing asthma in many older adults [1]. In fact, allergen avoidance strategies are considered "front line" for allergy control in the older adult population. Older individuals often spend more time indoors and live in older dwellings with older furniture that may have accumulated dust mites, cockroaches, and mold [8]. A deep cleaning of the home, upholstery, and drapes, removal of older carpeting, and placement of HEPA (high-efficiency particulate air) filters have the potential to dramatically reduce allergen exposure [8]. Mitigation strategies may provide further benefit as older adults can suffer with polypharmacy and side effects related to the concomitant use of asthma and allergy medications (anticholinergic effects, increased intraocular pressure, and impaired hepatic/renal metabolism) [8]. Environmental control strategies should be tailored to relevant allergen and irritant exposures based on the patient's environmental history. Household allergen levels are often related to the degree of housing deterioration and thus pose an important target for public health interventions to improve asthma control [9]. A 2012 study performed by O'Sullivan revealed that adults with asthma receive significant benefit from environmental remediation including repair of water leaks, pest extermination, flooring, and wall repair [9]. Water damage is especially noxious as it enhances the growth of many allergens, including cockroach, mold, house dust mite, and rodents [9]. As a result of the remediation efforts undertaken by O'Sullivan's team, adult asthmatics experienced increase peak expiratory flow rate (PEFR) by 38.6 liter/minute, decreased rate of ED visits by 1.67, and decreased hospitalization by 0.83 over the following 6–12 months [9]. All patients enrolled in the study dropped one class in asthma severity [9]. The paragraphs that follow provide detailed information regarding remediation and environmental control strategies that are especially important for many older adults with asthma.

Cockroach

The most common cockroach species present in the urban environment in the United States include German and American cockroaches. The major cockroach allergens are Bla g 1 (German) and Bla a 2 (American). Cockroach infestation is more commonly associated with a highly dense population, an urban environment, and low socioeconomic status [10]. Within homes, cockroaches are often found in kitchens as they are drawn to food and water [11]. At least 50% of low-income urban housing and 30% of suburban housing have clinically relevant levels of cockroach allergen [7]. The combination of cockroach sensitization and exposure is a frequent trigger of asthma-related morbidity, including hospitalization [11]. These allergens are carried on large particles, generally greater than 10 microns, which are less likely to remain airborne. Consequently, asthmatics sensitized to cockroach (and house dust mites) rarely recognize the temporal association between allergen exposure and symptoms. This is in contrast to those allergic to animal dander carried on smaller particles (less than 5 microns), where the temporal association is generally more obvious [4]. Multifaceted environmental interventions known as integrated pest management (IPM) (Table 11.1) can be implemented to reduce infestation. Implementation of these recommendations has been associated with dramatic reduction in cockroach allergen levels by 80–90% and improvement in asthmatic symptoms and quality of life [7]. While formal studies detailing the clinical benefit of IPM in older adults with asthma have not been undertaken, reduction in asthma-related morbidity has been observed in pediatric asthmatics when cockroach allergy levels are reduced by 50–90% [7]. Interventions include application of pesticides, of which gel form is preferred over aerosols to minimize pesticide exposure, sealing cracks, vigorous cleaning, and prompt disposal of food waste [7] (Table 11.2).

Table 11.1 Environmental Triggers for Asthma [11]

Exposure	Intervention for reduced exposure
Aeroallergens	Integrated pest management
	Aeroallergen avoidance techniques
	Repair of housing conditions
Infection	Annual influenza vaccination, consider high-dose option for those older than age 65 years
	Pneumococcal vaccination: Pneumovax, Prevnar
	Antiviral treatment within 48 hours of flu symptoms
Pollutants (indoor/ outdoor)	Tobacco cessation by patient/family members
	Regularly assess home ventilation systems
	Choose furnishings with low chemical emissions
	Minimize residential proximity to diesel exhaust
	Follow EPA AQI recommendations

Table 11.2 Aeroallergens and corresponding environmental control measures [11]

Aeroallergen	Environmental control recommendations
Cockroach	Keep kitchen clean/tidy
	Prompt washing of all dishes and cookware
	Keeping food in sealed containers
	Frequent disposal of trash
	Integrative pest management
	Extermination professional or use of gel bait
House dust mites	Maintain indoor relative humidity less than 45–50 °C
	Eradication of mite reservoirs: carpet, drapes, and upholstery
	Wash bedding weekly in hot water and hot dryer
	Vacuum carpets and rugs weekly with HEPA filter vacuum
	Use of impermeable encasements for pillows, mattress, and quilts
	Minimize dust collection on household objects
Mold	Limited use (if any) of humidifiers and vaporizers
	Dehumidifiers used in basement and other damp areas
	Control indoor humidity
	Remediation of water damage
	Clean nonporous surfaces with dilute bleach solution
Pets	Removal of pet from the home
	Keep pet out of the main living areas and bedroom
	HEPA filter air cleaners
	Wash pet regularly (twice per week as the benefit persists only 2–3 days)
	Removal of carpets and rugs
	Vacuum carpets and rugs weekly with HEPA filter vacuum
Rodents	Integrative pest management

House Dust Mite

House dust mites (HDM) are ubiquitous microscopic members of the arachnoid family that live in human dwellings and eat exfoliated human skin cells [11–13]. Their gut contains proteases that persist in feces and are thought to induce allergic sensitization and asthma. The two major HDM allergens, Der f 1 and Der p 1, come from the two most common dust mite species: *Dermatophagoides farinae* and *Dermatophagoides pteronyssinus*. HDM proliferation is favored by increased indoor humidity greater than 65% and warmer temperatures as they absorb water from their surrounding environment [13, 14]. HDM are rare in more arid climates. Similar to cockroach allergen, dust mite allergens travel on large particles (greater than 10 microns) and therefore settle quickly on surfaces. The highest concentrations of Der f 1 and Der p 1 are typically found in bedding, upholstered furniture, plush toys, and carpeting, as these surfaces harbor exfoliated human skin cells. HDM exposure is correlated to the degree of sensitization and airway inflammation that results from chronic exposure to small amounts of these large particles [13]. It is important for providers to recognize that clinical history from the patient will not provide evidence about the levels of HDM allergen in the home.

Decreasing exposure to HDM requires a multifaceted intervention approach addressing facilitative factors for proliferation and eradication of reservoirs [13]. Mitigation strategies to reduce exposure to house dust mites include reduction of indoor humidity, frequent washing of bed linens in hot water, use of allergen impermeable finely woven mattress and pillow encasements, and elimination of reservoirs through frequent vacuuming and/or removal of carpet and plush toys [10, 13] (Table 11.1). HDM rely on ambient moisture in the environment for growth and reproduction; therefore, keeping humidity at 45% or less is an important tenet for allergen control [10]. Elevated humidity for even 1.5 hours per day can allow mites to survive. If humidity is increased for 3 hours per day, mites are able to produce eggs [13]. Regular washing of bedding and clothing has been shown to effectively remove mite allergens and kill live mites through drowning and heat exposure [13]. It is generally recommended that fabric materials be kept to a minimum in the home [10]. Area rugs can be cleaned and dried in the sun, and HEPA-certified vacuum cleaners are recommended for decreasing HDM allergen burden in carpeting [10, 13]. While vacuum cleaners are effective at removing dust allergen in the form of fecal particles, they also disturb dust particles. It is therefore recommended that patients either wear a mask while vacuuming or refrain from entering the cleaned room for 20 minutes until disturbed particles have settled [10]. Live mites are rarely removed from carpet with the use of vacuums, as their foot pads allow them to remain adherent to a variety of surfaces [10]. Woven encasements with a mean pore size <10 micrometers should be utilized, as previous studies with live mites revealed their ability to permeate unwoven fabrics [10, 13]. Additionally, encasements prepared with unwoven fabrics are often contaminated with debris from mites and do not withstand repeated washing or use [10]. Physical measures for eradication including heating, freezing, and drying theoretically are helpful; however, no clinical trials to date have demonstrated benefit. No studies have specifically evaluated the above strategies in older adults; however, current guidelines and practice parameters advise that HDM-sensitized patients of any age with rhinitis and/or asthma minimize exposure to prevent development of symptoms [13].

Mold

More than 100,000 fungal species have been described, with greater than 80 indoor molds responsible for adverse health effects in humans [11, 15]. The International Union of Immunological Societies (IUIS) has determined that there are more than 111 fungal allergens implicated with human disease [15]. Fungal exposure has been associated with the development of asthma, the degree of asthma severity, and acute exacerbations in younger populations but has not been well studied in older asthmatics [7, 16]. Sensitivity to *Aspergillus fumigatus* has been associated with severe persistent asthma in adults [7, 16]. Exposure to high spores counts of *Alternaria alternata* has been associated with increased airway hyper-reactivity and severe asthma exacerbations, including sudden respiratory arrest and asthma-associated deaths [7, 16]. In one study, asthma deaths in Chicago were more than twice as high on days when there were more than 1000 *Alternaria* spores/M^3 [16]. Sensitivity to *Alternaria alternata* and *Cladosporium herbarum* has also been linked with development of asthma in children and persistence of asthma into adulthood [15]. Fungal spores have also been implicated in several cases of thunderstorm-induced asthma [16].

Mold spores are quite heterogeneous in regard to their size and shape, ranging from 2 to 250 microns, and therefore can penetrate any level of the respiratory tree [7, 14]. The most common offending molds include the outdoor species of *Cladosporium herbarum* and *Alternaria alternata* and the indoor species of *Aspergillus fumigatus* and *Penicillium notatum*, associated with indoor dampness [7, 14]. Outdoor molds can enter buildings through open windows and doors, on clothing surfaces and pet fur, and will proliferate indoors if conditions are suitable for growth [7, 17]. Concentrations of outdoor airborne fungi are highest in the late summer and early fall due to increased temperature and high dew point, with counts as high as 50,000 spores/M^3 during those months, and lowest in the winter at 50 spores/M^3 [16, 17]. Factors influencing the concentration of mold spores in the home include the age of the dwelling, the presence of a basement/crawl space, presence of water damage/leaks, use of humidifiers, and the condition of central heating, ventilation, and air-conditioning (HVAC) systems.

Use of HVAC systems with properly maintained filters has been shown to reduce transport of outdoor mold spores into homes [7]. The best predictors for indoor mold concentration are the outdoor concentration when windows are open and dampness in the home when windows are closed [16]. Several studies including systematic reviews, case-control studies, and the Institute of Medicine Report have linked indoor dampness with development of asthma [16]. Indoor molds are typically isolated from buildings that suffer from excessive moisture resulting in "water intrusion, inadequate ventilation, defective plumbing or other maintenance issues" [7]. Building materials prone to fungal attacks include organic materials containing cellulose, wood, jute, wallpaper, drywall, and cardboard [16]. Air sampling, moisture meters, and environmental history are all useful tools to identify moisture issues. Air sampling as a means to identify mold growth requires the use of indoor and outdoor samples for comparison [7, 12]. A previous study of fungal sensitization in West Virginia patients aged 8–78 years old revealed fungal sensitization based on skin testing ranged between 8% and 14%; this is comparable to the rate of fungal sensitization in German children at 8.3% [15]. Molds can cause symptoms through both IgE and non-IgE-mediated mechanisms; therefore, one does not need to be sensitized to fungi in order to become symptomatic with exposure [7, 17].

A Cochrane meta-analysis revealed that mitigation of mold damage in homes, schools, and offices decreased asthma-related symptoms and respiratory infections in adults [16, 18]. The best approach for mold eradication is multipronged with attention to resolution of enabling factors, removal of reservoirs, and prevention of dissemination from source to occupants [17]. The most effective strategy to prevent and reduce fungal growth is moisture control, with focus on water entry from the outside usually through cracks/holes in the foundation or walls, roofs, or windows. This also includes elimination of condensation that may occur on cold pipes and basement walls and elimination of water leakage from water pipes, drains, and faucets [17]. For patients with allergic asthma and sensitivity to fungal allergens, the use of HVAC with maintained filters can help reduce the transmission of outdoor

Table 11.3 Considerations for the performance of fungal assessment [20]

Considerations for the performance of fungal assessment by indoor environmental professional (IEP)
1. Occurrence of increased respiratory symptoms after home occupancy
2. The patient plans to reside in the home long term
3. The patient has control over the indoor environment to implement proposed interventions

fungal spores to the indoor environment [7]. Caution should be exercised when attempting to remove visible fungal growth. The National Institute of Occupational Safety and Health recommends wearing an N-95 mask and the use of a dilute chlorine-based bleach solution to remove fungi from nonporous surfaces [7]. Porous surfaces contaminated by fungal growth are unable to be cleansed due to mold penetration deep into the material [17]. While many issues related to fungal contamination and dampness can be remedied by the patient themselves, an indoor environmental professional (IEP) may be required. The Centers for Disease Control and Prevention recommends ensuring that the IEP has experience in mold eradication and adheres to the guidelines set forth by the Environmental Protection Agency or American Conference of Governmental Industrial Hygienists [7]. A professional fungal assessment should be considered if [19] the patient has lived in the home long enough for respiratory symptoms to occur; [1] symptoms occurred after occupying the home; [5] the patient is likely to remain in the home long enough to justify remediation; and [6] the patient has sufficient control of the environment to implement interventions [20] (Table 11.3).

Furry Pets

Although specific information regarding pet allergy in older adults is not available, pets can represent an important source of allergen exposure in atopic individuals of any age. According to market research done by the American Humane Association, approximately 62% of American families have a pet, the highest percentage of household pets worldwide [7, 11, 21]. In the general public, approximately 12% of individuals are sensitized to pet allergens, with slightly higher rates of sensitization in pet owners [7]. Approximately 17% of individuals with a cat are skin test positive to cat, and 5% of individuals with a dog are skin test positive to dog [21]. The allergens associated with cat and dog sensitivity can be isolated from saliva, sloughed skin particles, and hair follicles [7, 8]. The major allergens for cat include Fel d 1 (secretoglobulin), Fel d 2 (albumin), Fel d 3 (cystatin), Fel d 4 (lipocalin), Fel d 5 (IgA), Fel d 6 (IgM), Fel d 7 (lipocalin-Von Ebner's gland protein), and Fel d 8 (latherin) [22]. Fel d 1 is considered to be the major cat allergen as more than 90% of cat allergic patients are sensitized to this protein [21, 22]. All cats produce detectable levels to at least one or more of these clinically significant allergens, subsequently there are no confirmatory studies regarding the existence of hypoallergenic cats [21]. The degree of sensitivity to cat depends on which allergens a patient is sensitized to and which allergens are produced by the cat [22]. The major allergens for dog are Can f 1 (lipocalin), Can f 2 (lipocalin), Can f 3 (albumin), Can f 4 (odor-ant binding/prostatic kallikrein lipocalin), Can f 5 (trypsin like protease), and Can f 6 (lipocalin) [22]. Can f 2 has considerable cross-reactivity with Fel d 4, which explains the very frequent co-sensitization to both cats and dogs [22]. In compari-son to cat allergy, only 52% of dog-allergic patients are sensitive to Can f 1, with varying rates of sensitivity to the other major dog allergens [22]. Can f 3 is dog albumin and subsequently produced by all dogs, even hypoallergenic dog species [22]. In addition, previous studies have shown similar levels of allergen production between hypoallergenic and traditional dogs [21, 22].

Pet allergen exposure has been linked to poorer asthma outcomes and increased symptoms in sensitized adults [22]. Older asthmatics should be asked about the presence of a pet during their environmental history; however, absence of a pet in the home does not exclude clinically significant pet allergen exposure [12]. Furry pet allergen is adherent to a variety of surfaces including clothing, walls, and furni-ture. Given their small size, ranging from 2 to 10 microns, they remain airborne for a prolonged period of time [7, 11, 12]. The 2012 Practice Parameter Guidelines on furry animals recommends that exposure to offending pets be minimized in sensi-tized adult patients to reduce the likelihood of asthma development, asthma exacer-bations, and worsening of symptoms [22]. A prospective, non-randomized study found that pet removal in newly diagnosed pet allergic adults was associated with substantial reductions in asthma-controller medications [7]. It can take up to 6 months after removal of a pet for there to be significant reductions in allergen levels [21]. While avoidance is the most effective strategy for management of furry pet allergy, many pet owners are reluctant to remove their pet. In this case, patients should consider a multipronged approach to lessen pet allergen reservoirs, including keeping the pet out of the bedroom, washing the pet regularly, and use of HEPA-certified filters and vacuums [22]. Washing pets does diminish allergen presence in their fur, but the effect only persists for 2–3 days [4, 7, 21]. The use of HEPA filters has been associated with a 30–40% decrease in airborne cat allergen levels; how-ever, the filters do not remove pet allergen from settled dust, and corresponding improvements in asthma and allergic rhinitis symptoms have not been proven [7]. There is no evidence that owning "hypoallergenic" cats or dogs lowers the risk of pet-related asthma or rhinitis among allergic individuals.

Rodents

The impact of rodent allergy on older asthmatics has not specifically been studied; however, information from younger asthmatic populations has important implica-tions for older adults as well. Approximately 75–80% of US homes have detectable levels of mouse allergen [12]. Concentrations in inner city dwellings are 100- to 1000-fold higher than those in the suburbs [23]. Mus m 1, the major mouse allergen, can be isolated from mouse hair follicles and skin [24]. Similar to other furry animal allergens, Mus m 1 remains airborne for a prolonged period of time [12, 24]. Any evidence of infestation suggests clinically significant mouse allergen levels;

however, lack of infestation does not exclude the presence of mouse allergen in the home [12]. Several studies have revealed that sensitization to mouse allergen in children and adolescents is associated with a higher risk of asthma morbidity, with a linear dose-response relationship between mouse allergen concentrations and asthma-associated morbidity [25, 26]. Unfortunately, similar studies have not been replicated in older asthmatics. Mouse allergen levels can be reduced with the use of professional integrated pest management (IPM), utilizing a variety of interventions including pest traps, sealing holes/cracks that serve as rodent entry sites, and application of rodenticide [7, 12, 24]. There is an association between large reductions of rodent allergen levels (>50–75% reduction) and clinical improvement in asthma outcomes in inner-city pediatric asthmatics [7]. Rodents are a well-recognized cause of occupational rhinitis and asthma, which is important to keep in mind for older adults that are employed in biomedical research (Table 11.1).

Infections

Older asthmatics may be disproportionally impacted by infections as compared to younger adults; this is due to immune senescence, physiological changes that occur with age, and the potential for increased exposure to infection as a result of residence in facilities and grandchildren [8]. Immune senescence affects both innate and adaptive arms of the immune system through multiple mechanisms, including reduced mucociliary clearance, impairment of high-affinity antibody production, and thymic atrophy resulting in decreased naïve T-cell diversity [8]. These factors lead to an increased risk of respiratory infections in older adults, which could exacerbate asthma or even provoke the development of late-onset asthma [2]. The major impact of immune senescence is increased susceptibility to microbial infection, including viral and bacterial infections that can trigger asthma exacerbations in older adults [1]. Respiratory viral infection is a common culprit for asthma exacerbation, occurring in 70% of inpatients with an asthma exacerbation [27]. In a recent study by Likura, the cause of asthma exacerbation in adults ranging in age from 28 to 92 years (mean age 58) requiring inpatient admission was viral infection in 33.3%, bacterial infection in 18.8%, co-existing bacterial and viral infection in 18.8%, and no infection in 29.2% [27]. The most commonly encountered viruses include rhinovirus A/B/C (HRV), respiratory syncytial virus A (RSV), influenza A (IF), and human metapneumovirus. HRV induces asthma exacerbations due to its potential to induce a TH2 response [27]. Influenza A circulates annually across the United States from late fall to early spring and has been associated with serious illness and death in older adults and those with chronic medical conditions, such as asthma [27–29]. Influenza A increases asthma symptoms, rates of exacerbations, and complications including pneumonia [30]. Asthma was the most common underlying medical condition in patients hospitalized with H1N1 during the 2009 influenza pandemic [30]. RSV is being increasingly identified as a cause of intensive care unit admission with ventilator support. Higher levels of RSV are isolated from adults with any primary pulmonary disease, including asthma, residing in nursing home or long-term care facilities [31]. Patients are often exposed to viruses and allergens simultaneously, which synergistically increase the risk of an acute severe exacerbation [1]. In one study, infection with *Streptococcus pneumoniae* was the largest risk factor in adult asthma exacerbations requiring inpatient management [27]. Other common bacterial pathogens identified included *Haemophilus influenzae*, as well as atypical bacteria species such as *Chlamydophila pneumoniae* and *Mycoplasma pneumoniae* [27]. Compared to patients with non-infection-induced asthma exacerbations, patients with a detectable pathogen determined via nasopharyngeal viral/bacterial PCR and/or sputum culture were generally older, had later onset of asthma, were more likely to be nonatopic as assessed via fractional exhaled nitric oxide (FENO) level and total IgE, and had higher rates of comorbid sinusitis, tobacco exposure, and pneumonia [27].

Influenza and pneumococcal disease are vaccine-preventable infectious diseases that together are responsible for more than 260,000 hospitalizations and 40,000 deaths annually in the United States, with greater effects on older adults [32]. Vaccination is a proven, effective approach to help maintain immune responses and prevent infectious disease in older adults. Both annual influenza and routine pneumococcal vaccination are effective at preventing development of these infectious diseases in older adults, thus preventing deterioration of asthma control. Unfortunately, influenza vaccination rates remain far below the Healthy People 2020 objective of 90% in those older than age 18 years [1, 30, 32]. A Center for Disease Control (CDC) report in 2013 revealed that in the 2010–2011 season, only 50% of asthmatics had received annual influenza vaccination [30]. The CDC and CDC Advisory Committee on Immunization Practices recommends seasonal influenza vaccination to all individuals greater than 6 months of age without contraindication [28, 33]. While healthcare access is positively associated with improved influenza vaccination rates, the prevalence of asthma is negatively associated with vaccination in older adults, for unclear reasons [33]. Thus, vaccination remains an important target of care for older asthmatics to minimize exacerbations related to infection. For patients older than age 65, 2017–2018 CDC guidelines recommend any age-appropriate inactivated influenza vaccine (IIV) formulation, including standard dose (SD-IIV) or high-dose (HD-IIV), trivalent (IIV3) or quadrivalent (IIV4), unadjuvanted or adjuvated (aIIV3), or recombinant vaccine (RIV). There are no preferential recommendations for a specific vaccine [28]. Quadrivalent vaccines differ from trivalent in that each vaccine contains one virus from each of the two B influenza lineages (Victoria/Yamagata), whereas trivalent contain only one B influenza lineage [28]. Quadrivalent vaccines are therefore thought to provide better and broader protection against influenza B viruses; however, there is no preference for IIV3 or IIV4 in older adults [28]. High dose (HD-IIV3) has shown superior efficacy over standard dose (SD-IIV3) in patients greater than 65 years old [34]. This was measured by higher hemagglutinin-inhibition antibody (HAI) titers over two seasons, which implies improved viral protection [34]. Flublock, a recombinant, quadrivalent vaccine (RIV4) was shown to be more effective in reducing the PCR-confirmed influenza attack rates than SD-IIV4 in adults greater than age 50 [35]. Older patients vaccinated with RIV4 had a 30% reduced probability of influenza-like illness in comparison to those vaccinated with IIV4 [35]. Fluad (aIIV3) was shown to be more effective than unadjuvanted SD-IIV3 in patients older than age 65 [28]. Given the increased risk of illness, hospitalization, and death associated with influenza in older adults, there is much ongoing research evaluating the efficacy and effect of specific influenza vaccinations in this population. To date, studies have only compared the efficacy of HD-IIV3 (Fluzone), RIV4 (Flublock), and aIIV3 (Fluad) standard dose, inactivated vaccines. There are no data at this time comparing the efficacy or effectiveness of HD-IIV3, aIIV3, and RIV4 in older adults [28]. Spangnuolo et al. investigated the benefit of antiviral treatment over four influenza seasons when initiated within 48 hours of diagnosis. Antiviral treatment was found to reduce the overall risk of complications by 11% and led to lower healthcare utilization including hospitalization, emergency department visits, or physician visits as measured by claims data [29].

Pneumococcal disease is another leading cause of vaccine-preventable disease and death in older adults; this includes cases of pneumonia, meningitis, and bacteremia [36]. The CDC and CDC Advisory Committee on Immunization Practices recommends pneumococcal vaccination (Prevnar PCV13 and Pneumovax PPSV23) to all adults older than age 65 years. They recommend treatment with PCV13 for all adults whom have not previously received a dose with PPSV23 vaccination. Vaccination with PPSV23 should occur approximately 1 year after PCV13 vaccination or 5 years after previous PPSV23 vaccination [36]. In older asthmatic patients, early treatment with antibiotics, antivirals, steroids, and bronchodilators may be necessary to prevent asthma exacerbation in the setting of an acute respiratory infection.

Air Pollution

Older adults are particularly susceptible to the effects of both indoor and outdoor air pollutants. They may have greater exposure to indoor pollutants than younger individuals due to spending more time inside the home. Age-related decline in antioxidant defenses increases susceptibility to indoor and outdoor air pollutants as well [37]. Older asthmatics are at increased risk of hospital admissions and reduced lung function due to acute elevations in nitrogen dioxide, ozone, and particulate matter with diameters less than 2.5 μm (PM2.5) [38, 39]. Long-term residential exposure to traffic-related air pollutants has also been correlated with more poorly controlled asthma and decreased asthma-related quality of life in older asthmatics [11].

Indoor Air Pollutants

The most prevalent indoor air pollutant is tobacco smoke. It is well known that second-hand tobacco exposure can worsen asthma control and results in higher rates of ED visits for asthmatics of all ages [40]. Active tobacco smoke increases the severity of asthma and hinders the ability to gain symptom control. Second-hand tobacco exposure in the home also increases risks through contamination of the indoor environment and augmentation of allergic sensitization. Each half pack of cigarettes smoked in the home is estimated to contribute 4.0 micrograms/meter^3 of PM. Increased cotinine levels are also associated with increased prevalence of IgE sensitization to environmental allergens [14]. Based on hair nicotine levels, the impact of second-hand tobacco exposure may be especially pronounced in women [41]. The most effective means to reduce eliminate tobacco smoke exposure is smoking cessation either by the patient or close family members and caregivers [12]. HEPA devices may also reduce second-hand tobacco exposure homes where cessation has not been achieved [42].

Other relevant sources of indoor pollution include the use of cooking-related pollutants, pesticide sprays, cleaning materials that generate volatile organic compounds (VOCs), and furniture and building materials that emit aldehydes. Indoor air quality improvement measures are imperative for maintaining asthma control given that older adults spend a greater percentage of time indoors. Housing interventions that improve energy efficiency and reduce greenhouse gas emissions have been shown to result in changes in exposure to PM2.5 from indoor sources, resulting in decreased morbidity and mortality from asthma, cardiovascular disease, and lung cancer; the effects on cardiovascular disease and lung cancer are especially pronounced in older adults [43]. In an attempt to improve indoor air quality, patients should choose furniture with reduced chemical emissions and regularly assess their home ventilation systems. This includes regular opening of windows/doors to allow fresh air to enter and dilute possible harmful chemicals from furniture and construction. Patients may also consider implementing the use of a home HEPA-certified filtration system. These devices can significantly reduce particulate matter in homes as well as aeroallergens [42].

Outdoor Air Pollutants

Particulate matter (PM) is a mixture of solid and liquid particles of various sizes, shapes, and compositions suspended in the air. The size of PM determines their level of penetration into the respiratory tree and subsequent symptoms. Coarse PM ranges from 2.5 to 10 microns and can penetrate the airway at the level of the nasopharynx, oropharynx, larynx, trachea, and bronchi. Fine and ultrafine PM are defined as less than 2.5 and less than 0.1 microns in size, respectively, and can penetrate further into the airway reaching the bronchioles and alveoli [14]. Multiple studies have reported increased allergic symptoms, allergen sensitivity, and reduced lung function with higher exposure to PM, such as those living in close proximity to high-density traffic. Even brief exposure to outdoor pollution can induce bronchospasm, wheeze, chest tightness, and shortness of breath in susceptible patients [44]. Air pollution exposure can augment allergy-related symptoms; previous studies have shown an increase in allergen-related asthma exacerbations in response to PM. Older patients with asthma may be more susceptible to elevated levels of outdoor air pollutants, including nitric oxide, ozone, and particulates, due to age-related decline in response to oxidative stress. A study involving 104 asthmatics age 65 years and older revealed that mean daily residential exposure to ECAT (elemental carbon attributable to traffic) was associated with poorer asthma control in older patients, as measured by Asthma Control Questionnaire (ACQ) scores and exacerbation frequency. ECAT used in these studies was based on land use regression modeling to estimate the distribution of ultrafine particles release from diesel exhaust. Patients with an ECAT exposure level of 0.39 micrograms/m^3 or higher were three times more likely to need two or more courses of prednisone in the previous 12 months [45]. Subsequent investigation revealed that chronic exposure to higher ECAT levels was associated with poorer quality of life as measured by the AQLQ, and eosinophilic airway inflammation as measured in induced sputum [46, 47]. The authors therefore recommended that residential proximity to traffic exhaust be considered as part of the environmental history in patients over age 65 years old, and interventions to reduce this exposure be encouraged.

Patients can take action to minimize the effects of outdoor air pollution on lung health. The United States Environmental Protection Agency utilizes the AQI (air quality index) to report daily air quality levels based on measurement of ground level ozone, particle emission, carbon monoxide, and sulfur dioxide. The EPA has outlined specific recommendations based on the daily AQI level. When air quality reaches a certain threshold, asthmatic patients are recommended to reduce their time spent outside and avoid exertion and strenuous activity. Other hypothesized recommendations such as wearing a paper dust mask and consumption of antioxidants have failed to provide any clinically significant benefit [11]. Sustained clean air policies are likely to be the most effective means to reduce adverse health effects related to air pollutants in all age groups.

Conclusion

Many triggers, both allergic and non-allergic, can influence asthma control in older adults. Asthma exacerbations in older adults are often due to a variety of allergic and non-allergic triggers including indoor allergens, viral infections, and air pollutants (indoor and outdoor). An environmental history is key to identify potential triggers and targets for remediation. It is important for healthcare providers and patients to recognize and avoid potential triggers in order to maintain asthma control and reduce associated morbidity and mortality. Given that multiple types of exposures can play a role in poor asthma control in older adults, multifaceted interventions are generally more effective than isolated interventions. Given potential for increased susceptibility to infections that can precipitate asthma exacerbations, older asthmatics should also remain up to date on routine vaccinations including influenza and pneumococcal vaccinations [19, 28, 32, 34–36]. Further studies are needed regarding intervention strategies that will reduce asthma-related morbidity and mortality related to aeroallergens, air pollution, and infectious exposures in this age group.

References

1. Yanez A, Cho SH, Soriano JB, et al. Asthma in the elderly: what we know and what we have yet to know. World Allergy Organ J. 2014;7:8.
2. Agondi RC, Andrade MC, Takejima P, et al. Atopy is associated with age at asthma onset in elderly patients. J Allergy Clin Immunol Pract. 2017;43:451–463.
3. Cardona V, Guilarte M, Luengo O, et al. Allergic disease of the elderly. Clinical Transl Allergy. 2011;1:11.
4. Custovic A, Simpson A. The role of inhalant allergens in allergic airways disease. J Investig Allergol Clin Immunol. 2012;22(6):393–401.
5. Rogers L, Cassino C, Berger KI, et al. Asthma in the elderly- cockroach sensitization and severity of airway obstruction in elderly nonsmokers. Chest. 2002;122(5):1580–6.
6. Busse PJ, Lushlurchachai L, Sampson HA. Perennial allergen-specific IgE levels amount innercity elderly asthmatics. J Asthma. 2010;47(7):781–5.
7. Ahluwalia SK, Matsui EC. Indoor environmental interventions for furry pet allergens, pest allergens and mold: looking to the future. J Allergy Clin Immunol Pract. 2018;6(1):9–19.
8. Calhoun KH. Allergy in the geriatric population. Curr Opin Otolaryngol Head Neck Surg. 2015;23:235–9.
9. O'Sullivan MM, Brandfield J, Hoskote SS, et al. Environmental improvements brought by the legal interventions in the homes of poorly controlled inner-city adult asthmatic patients: a proof of concept study. J Asthma. 2012;49(9):911–7.
10. Wilson JM, Platts-Mills TAE. Home environmental interventions for house dust mite. J Allergy Clin Immunol Pract. 2018;6(1):1–7.
11. Gautier C, Charpin D. Environmental triggers and avoidance in the management of asthma. J Asthma Allergy. 2017;10:47–56.
12. Matsui EC, Abramson SL, Sandel MT. Indoor environmental control practices and asthma management. Pediatrics. 2016;138:e1–e11.
13. Portnoy J, Miller JD, Williams B, et al. Environmental assessment and exposure control of dust mites: a practice parameter. Ann Allergy Asthma Immunol. 2013;111:465–507.
14. Singh M, Hays A. Indoor and outdoor allergies. Prim Care Clin Office Pract. 2016;43:451–63.
15. Brochers DH, Chang C, Gershwin ME. Mold and human health: a reality check. Clin Rev Allerg Immunol. 2017;52:305–22.
16. Baxi SN, Portnoy JM, Larenas-Linnemann D, Phipatanakul W. Exposure and health effects of Fungi on humans. J Allergy Clin Immunol Pract. 2016;4(3):396–404.
17. Portnoy JM, Jara D. Mold allergy revisited. Ann Allergy Asthma Immunol. 2015;114:83–9.
18. Sauni R, Verbeek JH, Utti J, et al. Remediating buildings damaged by dampness and mould for preventing or reducing respiratory tract symptoms, infections and asthma. Cochrane Database Syst Rev. 2015;(2):CD00787.
19. Scichilone N, Pedone C, Battaglia S, et al. Diagnosis and management of asthma in the elderly. Eur J Intern Med. 2014;25:336–242.
20. Chew GL, Horner E, Kennedy K. Procedures to assist health care providers to determine when home assessments for potential Mold exposure are warranted. J Allergy Clin Immunol Pract. 2016;4(3):417–22.
21. Butt A, Rashid D, Lockey RF. Do hypoallergenic cats and dogs exist? Ann Allergy Asthma Immunol. 2012;108:74–6.
22. Portnoy J, Kennedy K, Sublett J. Environmental assessment and exposure control: a practice parameter- furry animals. Ann Allergy Asthma Immunol. 2012, 108(4):223e1–223e15.
23. Cohn RD, Arbes SJ Jr, Yin M, et al. National prevalence and exposure for risk of mouse allergen in US households. J Allergy Clin Immunol. 20014;113(6):1167–71.
24. Phipatanakul W, Matsui E, Portnoy J, et al. Environmental assessment and exposure reduction of rodents: a practice parameter. Ann Allergy Asthma Immunol. 2012;109:375–87.

25. Ahuwalia SK, Peng RD, Breysse PN, et al. Mouse allergen is the major allergen of public health relevance in Baltimore City. J Allergy Clin Immunol. 2013;132:830–5.
26. Torjusen E, Diette GB, Breysse PN. Dose-response relationships between mouse allergen exposure and asthma morbidity among urban children and adolescents. J Allergy Clin Immunol. 2013;23:2680274.
27. Likura M, Hojo M, Koketsu R. The importance of bacterial and viral infections associated with adult asthma exacerbations in clinical practice. PLoS One. 2015;10:1–10.
28. Grohskopf LA, Sokolow LZ, Broder KR, Walter EB, Fry AM, Jernigan DB. Prevention and control of seasonal influenza with vaccines: recommendations of the advisory committee on immunization practices- United States, 2017–2018 influenza season. MMWR Recomm Rep. 2018;67(3):1–20. https://doi.org/10.15585/mmwr.rr6703a1.
29. Spagnuolo PH, Zhang M, Xu Y, Han J, Liu S, Liu J, Lichtveld M, Shi L. Effects of antiviral treatment on influenza-related complications over four influenza seasons: 2006-2010. Curr Med Res Opin. 2016;32(8):1399–407.
30. King M, Lu PJ, O'Halloran A, Ding H. Vaccination coverage among persons with asthma-United States, 2010–2011 influenza season. MMWR Morb Mortal Wkly Rep. 2013;62(48):973–8.
31. Binder W, Thorensen J, Borcuzk P. RSV in adult ED patients: do emergency providers consider RSV as an admission diagnosis. Am J Emerg Med. 2017;35:1162–5.
32. Michaelidis CL, Zimmerman RK, Nowalk MP, Smith KJ. Cost-effectiveness of programs to eliminate disparities in elderly vaccination rates in the United States. BMC Public Health. 2014;14:718.
33. Chiu APY, Dushoff J, Yu D, He D. Patterns of influenza vaccination coverage in the United States from 2009–2015. Int J Infect Dis. 2017;65:122–7.
34. DiazGranados CA, Dunning AJ, Kimmel M, et al. Efficacy of high dose versus standard-dose influenza vaccine in older adults. N Engl J Med. 2014;371(7):635–45.
35. Dunkle LM, Izikson R, Patriarca P, Goldenthal KL, et al. Efficacy of recombinant influenza vaccine in adults 50 years of age or older. N Engl J Med. 2017;376(25):2427–36.
36. Tomczyk S, Bennett NM, Stoecker C, et al. Use of 13-valent pneumococcal conjugate vaccine and 23-valent pneumococcal polysaccharide vaccine among adults aged >65 years: recommendations of the advisory committee on immunization practices. MMWR Morb Mortal Wkly Rep. 2014;63(37):822–5.
37. Ciencewicki J, Trivedi S, Kleeberger SR. Oxidants and the pathogenesis of lung diseases. J Allergy Clin Immunol. 2008;122(3):456–68. Quiz 469–470.
38. Anderson HR, Atkinson RW, Bremner SA, Marston L. Particulate air pollution and hospital admissions for cardiorespiratory diseases: are the elderly at greater risk? Eur Respir J Suppl. 2003;40:39s–46s.
39. Ko FM, Tam W, Wong TW, et al. Effects of air pollution on asthma hospitalization rates in different age groups in Hong Kong. Clin Exp Allergy. 2007;37:1312–9.
40. Rayens MK, Burkhart PV, Zhang M, et al. Reduction in asthma-related emergency department visits after implementation of a smoke-free law. J Allergy Clin Immunol. 2008;122(3):537–41.
41. Balmes JR, Cisternas M, Quinlan PJ, Trupin L, Lurmann FW, Katz PP, Blanc PD. Annual average ambient particulate matter exposures estimates, measured home particulate matter, and hair nicotine are associated with respiratory outcomes in adults with asthma. Environ Res. 2014;129:1–10.
42. Batterman S, Du L, Mentz G, et al. Particulate matter concentrations in residences: an intervention study evaluating stand-alone filters and air conditioners. Indoor Air. 2012;22(3):235–52.
43. Milner J, Chalabi Z, Vardoulakis S, Wilkinson P. Housing interventions and health: quantifying the impact of indoor particles on mortality and morbidity with disease recovery. Environ Int. 2015;81:73–9.
44. Jiang XQ, Mei XD, Feng D. Air pollution and chronic airway diseases: what should people know and do? J Thorac Dis. 2016;8(1):E31–40.

45. Epstein TG, Ryan PH, LeMasters GK, et al. Poor asthma control and exposure to traffic pollutants and obesity in older adults. Ann Allergy Asthma Immunol. 2012;108(6):423–8.
46. Kannan JA, Bernstein DI, Bernstein CK, et al. Significant predictors of poor quality of life in older asthmatics. Ann Allergy Asthma Immunol. 2015;115(3):198–204.
47. Epstein TG, Kesavalu B, Bernstein CK, et al. Chronic traffic pollution exposure is associated with eosinophilic, but not Neutrophilic inflammation in older adult asthmatics. J Asthma. 2013;50(9):983–9.

Novel and Alternative Therapies for Asthma in Older Adults

12

Dharani K. Narendra, Ali Cheema, and Nicola A. Hanania

Introduction

Worldwide estimates suggest that 617 million (8.5%) people were 65 years of age and older in 2016, and this number is projected to increase to include 17% of the population (1.6 billion) by 2050 [1, 2]. The current prevalence of asthma in patients above 65 years of age is estimated to be in the range of 4.5–12.7% [3, 4]. This is also estimated to increase dramatically in the near future. Asthma in this population is associated with higher morbidity and mortality than asthma in younger patients. Two phenotypes of asthma exist in the older population: long-standing asthma (LSA) and late onset asthma (LOA) (see Phenotypes Chapter). Several challenges in the management of asthma in older adults exist, and conventional therapies often fail to control the disease in this population [5].

Management of coexisting comorbidities as well as improving adherence to management plans are of extreme importance to ensure appropriate response to therapy [6, 7]. In selected populations, alternative therapies may be appropriate. Our improved understanding of the immunopathology of asthma in such patients has allowed the identification of several potential targets for novel therapies.

Novel Pharmacologic Targets

Biologic Agents

There has been a giant leap in the use of biologics in severe asthma over the last decade. Indeed, several agents are now approved by US Food and Drug Administration (FDA) for use in severe allergic and eosinophilic asthma; however,

D. K. Narendra · A. Cheema · N. A. Hanania (✉)
Pulmonary and Critical Care Medicine, Baylor College of Medicine, Houston, TX, USA
e-mail: Narendra@bcm.edu; Ali.Cheema@bcm.edu; hanania@bcm.edu

© Springer Nature Switzerland AG 2019
T. E. G. Epstein, S. M. Nyenhuis (eds.), *Treatment of Asthma in Older Adults*,
https://doi.org/10.1007/978-3-030-20554-6_12

data on their use in older adults are still emerging. A summary of biologics currently approved for treatment of severe asthma is listed in Table 12.1 and detailed below.

Targeting IgE (Omalizumab)

Omalizumab is a recombinant humanized IgG1 monoclonal antibody to IgE and was the first biological agent approved by FDA in 2003 as an add-on therapy for moderate-to-severe persistent allergic asthma in patients aged 6 and above inadequately controlled with high doses of inhaled corticosteroid therapy. Omalizumab acts by binding to circulating IgE and prevents its interaction with the high-affinity IgE receptor FC€RI, forming immune complexes, which are cleared by the hepatic reticuloendothelial system. This prevents IgE from activating mast cells and basophils and thereby interrupting the allergic cascade. To be a candidate for such therapy, a patient must demonstrate an elevated serum IgE level and either a positive allergen skin test or serum allergen-specific IgE test to perennial allergens. Omalizumab is administered by subcutaneous injection every 2–4 weeks in a dose that is determined by body weight and the levels of serum IgE.

Pooled data from seven randomized controlled studies with 4308 patients demonstrated that omalizumab reduced annual exacerbations by 38% and emergency department visits by 47%, and reduced use of systemic corticosteroids by 43% [8]. Patients with more severe asthma had the most benefit, which persists up to 2 years after stopping the medication. The response to omalizumab is more pronounced in patients with more severe disease, and in those with elevated blood eosinophils and exhaled nitric oxide levels (FeNO) [9]. More recently, emerging data support the beneficial effects of omalizumab in reducing viral-induced asthma exacerbations which may reflect a possible effect on viral clearance [10–12]. Omalizumab is generally well tolerated; however, anaphylaxis has been reported 1 or 2 per 1000 patients, with 70% occurring within first 2 hours after the injection [13]. Thus, it is recommended that all patients be educated about this potential side effect and prescribed epinephrine auto-injectors.

A retrospective study evaluated long-term effects of omalizumab by age in patients with asthma. One hundred five patients were administered omalizumab for a year [14]. They were divided into three age groups: 18–39, 40–64, and ≥65 years. Older patients had more comorbidities and were more obese. Following treatment, all three groups had reduced inhaled corticosteroid dose, improved asthma control test (ACT score), and similar improvement in $FEV_1\%$ predicted. Furthermore, omalizumab reduced asthma exacerbations significantly, although the percent of exacerbation-free patients was higher in younger ages (76.9%) compared to middle-aged patients (49.2%) and older adults (29%), $p = 0.049$ [10]. Several other small studies have shown that omalizumab is a well-tolerated and effective therapy for older adults with severe allergic asthma [15, 16].

In summary, omalizumab is recommended for older adult patients with severe allergic asthma who remain uncontrolled despite inhaled corticosteroids and other controller therapies.

Table 12.1 Target and efficacy of approved biologic therapies for asthma

Target	Drugs	Dosage	Route and frequency of administration	Target patient population	Clinical outcomes	Biomarkers identifying responders	Response in older patients
IgE	Omalizumab	150–375 mg[a]	S.C. Q 2 or 4 weeks[a]	Allergic asthma	↓ Exacerbations ↓ Hospitalizations ↓ ICS dose	FeNO Blood eosinophils Serum Periostin	Safe and effective
IL-5	Mepolizumab	100 mg	S.C. Q 4 weeks[b]	Eosinophilic asthma	↓ Exacerbations ↓ Oral glucocorticoid use	Blood eosinophils	Safe and effective
	Reslizumab	3 mg/Kg	I.V. Q 4 weeks[b]	Eosinophilic asthma	↓ exacerbations ↑ FEV₁	Blood eosinophils	Safe and effective
IL5Rα	Benralizumab	30 mg	S.C. Q 4 weeks X 3 and then Q 8 weeks[b]	Eosinophilic asthma	↓ Exacerbations ↑ FEV₁ ↓ Oral glucocorticoid use	Blood eosinophils	Safe and effective
IL-4Rα	Dupilumab	200 mg, 300 mg	S.C. Q 2 weeks[c]	Eosinophilic asthma	↓ Exacerbations ↑ FEV₁ ↓ Oral glucocorticoid use	Blood eosinophils FeNO	Safe and effective

S.C subcutaneous, *Q* every, *ICS* inhaled corticosteroids, *FEV1* forced expiratory volume in 1 second, *FeNO* fractional exhaled nitric oxide
[a]based on weight and total IgE level
[b]In clinic administration
[c]Initial dose 400 or 600 mg, home administration

Targeting Interleukin (IL)-5

Eosinophils are dominant effector cells in asthma, and their activation leads to airway injury, mucus hypersecretion, and bronchial hyper-responsiveness. Immune system studies have shown IL-5 to be involved in eosinophilic activation in the airway with upregulation in response to allergen exposure, an effect that is decreased in the setting of systemic steroids [17]. IL-5 is an effector cytokine that has a major effect on eosinophil recruitment and maturation. Therefore, blocking IL-5 and its activity is a very important target in managing severe eosinophilic asthma.

Mepolizumab

Mepolizumab is a monoclonal antibody to IL-5, which has been approved by the FDA and National Institute for Health and Care Excellence (NICE) as an add-on, maintenance treatment of severe eosinophilic asthma in patients who are aged 12 or older. It is administered monthly by subcutaneous injection.

In clinical trials, mepolizumab demonstrated a significant reduction of asthma exacerbations in patients with severe asthma who have high blood eosinophil counts (eosinophil count $\geq 300/\mu L$). Pavord and colleagues conducted a multicenter, double-blind placebo-controlled trial (DREAM) at 81 centers from 12 countries, including 621 patients who were randomized to three different strengths of mepolizumab [18]. The rate of clinically significant exacerbations was significantly reduced with mepolizumab (1.24/year in the 75 mg mepolizumab group, 1.46/year in the 250 mg mepolizumab, and 1.15/year in the 750 mg mepolizumab group compared to 2.4/year in the placebo group). Ortega and colleagues conducted another large trial on mepolizumab as adjunctive therapy in patients with severe asthma (MENSA) in which they randomized 576 patients with recurrent asthma exacerbations with evidence of eosinophilic inflammation despite high-dose inhaled glucocorticoids to one of three study groups [19]. Patients were randomized to either mepolizumab 75 mg intravenous or 100 mg subcutaneous or placebo subcutaneous every 4 weeks for 32 weeks. Screening criteria included patients with baseline blood eosinophils ≥ 150 cells/μL at screening or ≥ 300 cells/μL within 12 months of enrollment. Patients enrolled in this study included those between 12 and 82 years of age. The primary outcome of this study was asthma exacerbation, which was reduced by 47% (95% CI, 28–60) among patients receiving intravenous (IV) mepolizumab and 53% (95% CI: 36–65) among patients receiving subcutaneous mepolizumab compared to placebo (p <0.001). Furthermore, there were also significantly reduced emergency department visits, improvement in lung function (FEV_1), and quality of life measured by SGRQ total scores. Mepolizumab was evaluated in 80 elderly patients who were ≥ 65 years of age in subanalysis of MENSA trial [20]. Post-hoc analysis showed a 76% reduction in clinically significant exacerbations over the 32-week treatment period with mepolizumab compared with placebo (p <0.001). The quality of life measured by SGRQ was better in older patients compared to placebo, while safety profile and asthma control (ACQ-5) were similar in both groups.

In the SIRIUS trial, mepolizumab was evaluated in patients with severe eosinophilic asthma requiring oral glucocorticoids despite being on high-dose inhaled therapy [21]. One hundred thirty-five patients were randomized to mepolizumab (100 mg) versus placebo for 24 weeks. Mepolizumab was 2.39 times more likely to reduce oral steroid use compared to placebo (95% CI, 1.25–4.56, $p = 0.008$). At the end of the study, mepolizumab reduced oral glucocorticoid use by 50% compared to no reduction in the placebo group. The mepolizumab group had also a relative reduction in the annualized rate of exacerbations by 32%. The safety profile was similar in both groups. The benefits of mepolizumab on decreasing exacerbation rates and reducing corticosteroid use persisted after 1-year of follow-up.

Combining all three major trials, common adverse events included headache (19%), injection site reaction (8%), backpain and fatigue (5% each), and two patients developed herpes zoster. Because of its rare occurrence in these clinical trial population, the risk of herpes zoster infection in older patients with asthma treated with mepolizumab remains unknown and should be evaluated in future real-life studies. In the long-term safety and efficacy study of mepolizumab in patients with severe eosinophilic asthma, COLUMBA study, patients were followed for an average of 3.5 years to a maximum 4.5 years [22]. Mepolizumab decreased exacerbation rates by 61% (95% CI: 0.60–0.78), with consistent reduction in exacerbation rates per year over the study period. There was also a sustained and durable pharmacodynamic effect over time with no evidence of decreasing efficacy [23].

In summary, mepolizumab is considered safe in the use of older adult patients with uncontrolled severe persistent asthma with a blood eosinophil count more than 150 cells/µL. Herpes zoster vaccination may be considered 3–4 weeks before starting mepolizumab therapy.

Reslizumab

Reslizumab is a humanized, IgG4 monoclonal anti-IL-5 with a high affinity for the alpha subunit and blocks IL-5-mediated proliferation and neutralizes its effect [24]. An initial proof of concept pilot study by Kips et al. with 32 subjects showed that reslizumab was effective in reducing blood and sputum eosinophil counts at a dose of 1 mg/kg administered IV [25]. Although this study was not powered to detect clinical efficacy, in the subgroup of patients with raised eosinophil counts, there was a tendency for these patients to have an increase in FEV_1. This illustrates that reslizumab is safe and effective at reducing eosinophils and, importantly, that it may be necessary to select patients with residual eosinophilia to optimize its effect.

Castro et al. conducted the first large phase IIb study of reslizumab in a multi-center, randomized, double-blind, placebo-controlled trial ($n = 106$) [26]. The clinical efficacy of reslizumab administered IV (3 mg/kg, 4 weekly) was assessed by comparing Asthma Control Questionnaire (ACQ scores) and lung function in the treatment group versus the placebo group. Enrolled patients had confirmed airway reactivity, induced eosinophil sputum counts of ≥3%, and were on a high-dose ICS and a second controller. Reslizumab significantly reduced eosinophil numbers in sputum and improved lung function (FEV_1 baseline change was 0.18 L in the treatment group and − 0.08 L in the placebo group, $p = 0.002$). ACQ scores showed a trend toward better asthma control in the treatment group, and this was significant in the subgroup analysis of patients with nasal polyps. This study was encouraging as it clearly demonstrated significant benefit in those patients who had refractory eosinophilic asthma.

Two additional Phase III studies were conducted with the primary endpoint of frequency of clinical asthma exacerbations (CAE), defined as symptoms requiring oral steroids or at least doubling of ICS. These studies also looked at secondary endpoints of FEV_1, ACQ-7 asthma control score, Asthma Quality of Life Questionnaire (AQLQ) score, rescue use of short-acting bronchodilators, and blood eosinophil counts during the 52-week treatment phase, adjudicated by an independent review panel. Results showed a statistically significant decreased incidence of CAE in patients on reslizumab compared with placebo. This benefit extended to exacerbations requiring oral corticosteroids, thus providing evidence for the steroid-sparing effect of this therapy. Additionally, there were significant improvements in FEV_1, ACQ-7, Asthma Symptom Utility Index (ASUI), and Asthma Quality of Life Questionnaire (AQLQ) scores with reslizumab treatment, reduction in rescue short-acting beta 2-agonist use, and falls in blood eosinophils. Hospital admission rates were decreased and there was about a 20% absolute reduction in exacerbations over 1 year in patients on reslizumab compared to placebo [27]. Subsequent post-hoc analysis of the two Phase III studies by Brusselle et al. suggested that late-onset asthma (after the age of 40 years) responded better than the early-onset disease [28].

Bjermer et al. assessed a reslizumab dose-comparison study in a similar refractory asthma population over 16 weeks, with FEV_1 as the primary outcome [29]. They found that FEV_1 was significantly higher compared to placebo when dosed at 3 mg/kg compared to 0.3 mg/kg, without an increase in side effect profile. The authors concluded that the most effective dose was 3 mg/kg with a minimal side effect profile.

Reslizumab was evaluated in 122 patients who were 65 years and older with asthma in two 52-week exacerbation studies and two 16-week lung function studies. No overall differences in safety or effectiveness were observed between these patients and younger patients. Based on available data, no adjustment of the dosage of reslizumab in the older population is necessary.

In summary, these studies show that reslizumab is effective in patients with severe asthma and an eosinophil count of ≥ 400 cells/μL for an age range of 12–75 years. Furthermore, a dose of 3.0 mg/kg IV showed the most pronounced effect without an increase in adverse events (AEs). The most common AEs included: headache, upper respiratory infection, and nasopharyngitis. In addition, patients were less likely to discontinue treatment due to AEs in the reslizumab group compared to placebo [30].

Benralizumab

In contrast to mepolizumab and reslizumab, which are antibodies targeting IL-5 directly, benralizumab targets IL-5Rα which is the IL-5 receptor expressed on eosinophils and basophils in lung tissue and bone marrow, and leads to more complete depletion of eosinophils in lung tissue. Targeting IL-5 leads to upregulation of IL-5Rα expression and increased local production of IL-5 competing with

mepolizumab. By blocking IL-5Rα, benralizumab inhibits IL-5 binding independent of ligand and blocks downstream cell signaling. In addition, it also leads to
antibody-directed, cell-mediated cytotoxicity of eosinophils and basophils, thus
depleting IL-5Rα-expressing cells [31].

In a Phase 1 study evaluating the safety of benralizumab and its effect on eosinophil count, investigators demonstrated that there was no difference in adverse events
between treatment and placebo group but decrease of about 62% in airway mucosal
eosinophils, 18% in sputum, and 100% in blood by day 28 after single IV dose [32].
However, the effect was more pronounced in subjects who were given a subcutaneous formulation of benralizumab [33]. Nowak and colleagues investigated the utility of single dose of benralizumab in the Emergency Department (ED) setting for
patients with frequent asthma exacerbation defined as greater than one exacerbation
in past year [34]. Benralizumab decreased the asthma exacerbation rate by 49%, and
the exacerbations resulting in hospitalization rate by 60% over 12 weeks compared
to placebo. Authors concluded that one dose of benralizumab reduced the rate and
severity of asthma exacerbations over 12 weeks in subjects who presented to ED
with acute asthma [34]. In a phase 2b dose-ranging study, benralizumab efficacy
seemed to be enhanced for patients with blood eosinophil counts exceeding 300
cells per μL [35].

Two Phase 3 studies assessed the safety and efficacy of benralizumab in severe
asthma [36, 37]. The CALIMA trial involved 303 sites in 11 countries enrolling
patients aged 12–75 years with severe asthma uncontrolled with medium- to high-
dose inhaled corticosteroids plus long-acting β_2-agonists (ICU + LABA) with 2 or
more exacerbations in the previous year [36]. Patients were stratified based on blood
eosinophils either greater or less than 300 cells per μL and then randomized 1:1 to
receive 56 weeks of benralizumab 20 mg every 4 weeks (Q4W), benralizumab 30 mg
every 8 weeks (Q8W after first 3 doses 4 weeks apart), or placebo. Benralizumab
resulted in a significantly reduced rate of annual asthma exacerbations in the Q4W
(rate 0.60 [95% CI 0.48–0.74]) and Q8W (rate 0.66 [95% CI 0.54–0.82]) groups
compared to placebo (rate 0.93 [95% CI 0.77–1.12]). Benralizumab also significantly improved prebronchodilator FEV_1 and total asthma symptom score (Q8Wonly).
In the SIROCCO trial [37], a multicenter, placebo-controlled Phase 3 trial at 374
sites in 17 countries, patients were randomized 1:1:1 and stratified based on blood
eosinophils count (more than or less than 300 cells/μL) to two doses of benralizumab
(30 mg every 4 weeks or every 8 weeks, first 3 doses administered every 4 weeks)
versus placebo for 48 weeks. Compared to placebo, benralizumab reduced the annual
asthma exacerbation rate over 48 weeks (Q4W group rate 0.55, 95% CI 0.42–0.71,
$p < 0.0001$; and Q8W rate 0.49, 0.37 to 0.64; $p < 0.0001$). There was a significant
improvement in prebronchodilator FEV1 at week 48 compared to placebo. Asthma
symptoms were better in the Q8W regimen (least square mean difference, −0.25,
95% CI: −0.45 to −0.06), but not with Q4W regimen (−0.08, 95% CI: −0.27–0.12).
The most common adverse events were nasopharyngitis and worsening asthma, both
of which were equal in frequency compared to the control group.

Nair et al. conducted the ZONDA trial where 220 patients underwent randomization to two benralizumab dosing regimens: 30 mg administered subcutaneously

either every 4 weeks or every 8 weeks, with the first 3 doses administered every 4 weeks, or placebo [38]. The two benralizumab dosing regimens significantly reduced the median oral glucocorticoid use by 75% from baseline, while placebo only reduced use by 25% ($p < 0.001$). There was a significant reduction in the annual exacerbation rate with both doses of benralizumab compared to placebo. No significant change in FEV1 was noted, and adverse events were similar in both groups.

Based on population pharmacokinetic analysis, age did not affect benralizumab clearance. Of the total number of patients in clinical trials of benralizumab, 13% ($n = 320$) were 65 and older, while 0.4% ($n = 9$) were 75 and older. No overall differences in safety or effectiveness were observed between these patients and younger patients, and other reported clinical experience has not identified differences in responses between older and younger patients, but greater sensitivity of some older individuals cannot be ruled out.

In summary, the above studies illustrate the efficacy and safety of benralizumab for patients with severe asthma and elevated eosinophils, which are uncontrolled by high-dose ICS plus LABA, and provide support for benralizumab to be an additional treatment option in this patient population [30, 37].

Targeting IL-4/IL-13 (Dupilumab)

Dupilumab is a fully human monoclonal antibody directed against IL-4Rα, which inhibits IL-4/IL-13 signaling and thus downregulates type-2 airway inflammation. By binding the IL-4 receptor, dupilumab inhibits its activation by IL-4 and IL-13, thereby blocking downstream signal transduction and blunting the allergic response [31]. Dupilumab is approved for the treatment of atopic dermatitis, moderate-to-severe persistent eosinophilic asthma, and oral corticosteroid-dependent asthma.

In a Phase 2 trial conducted in patients with moderate-to-severe asthma on ICS and LABA with a high eosinophil profile, the rate of asthma exacerbations was 6% in the dupilumab group compared with 44% in placebo group when patients de-escalated their maintenance inhalers [39]. Other parameters that improved in the dupilumab group included: morning asthma symptom score, ACQ-5 score, use of albuterol, and nocturnal awakenings. Subsequent Phase III trials evaluated the long-term safety and efficacy of dupilumab in moderate-to-severe asthma who had a history of at least one asthma exacerbation in the past year [40, 41]. Investigators randomly assigned patients aged ≥12 years ($n = 1902$, Adults 1795) with uncontrolled asthma to receive subcutaneous dupilumab 200–300 mg every 2 weeks or matched placebo for 52 weeks. Results showed that severe asthma exacerbations were reduced by 47% in the treatment group compared to placebo. This reduction in asthma exacerbations was 65% in patients with uncontrolled asthma and blood eosinophil count ≥300 ml/μL and FeNO ≥25 ppb. In contrast, a poorer response was observed in patients with ≤150 eosinophils/μ and FeNO <25 ppb. Additionally, at 12 weeks, FEV_1 increased by 0.32 liters (L) in the treatment group compared to 0.14 L in the placebo group. Four percent of patients on dupilumab had increased level of eosinophils compared with 0.6% of patients in the placebo group. Rabe et al. investigated and published the safety and efficacy of dupilumab in glucocorticoid-dependent severe asthma [41]. Investigators randomly assigned 210 patients with oral corticosteroid-dependent asthma to receive add-on dupilumab 300 mg or placebo every two weeks for 24 weeks. Glucocorticoids were initially adjusted before randomization for symptom control and then adjusted downward from week 4 to week 20, with a stable dose for the last 4 weeks. Primary outcome results showed that the oral corticosteroid dose was decreased 70% in the dupilumab group compared with 42% in placebo group. Nearly 50% of patients in the treatment group completely discontinued oral corticosteroids, compared with 25% in placebo group. Secondary outcome results showed that despite a greater reduction in steroid dose in the treatment group, the rate of asthma exacerbations in the treatment group was 59% lower than in the placebo group, and FEV_1 was 0.22 L higher than in the placebo group. These results again were more pronounced for patient with eosinophil counts ≥ 300 cells/μL. Treatment was well tolerated with side effects including injection site reactions and increased transient blood eosinophilia in the treatment group.

In summary, data from Phase 2 and 3 studies confirm the efficacy and safety of dupilumab in severe T2 high asthma. Dupilumab can significantly reduce asthma exacerbations and improve lung function (increasing FEV_1), as well as reduce the dose of oral corticosteroids, in patients with moderate-to-severe allergic asthma. Additionally, it is the first biologic agent to show benefits in patients with severe corticosteroid-dependent asthma, regardless of blood eosinophil level [33].

Macrolides

Uncontrolled asthma despite maintenance therapy carries significant morbidity with frequent exacerbations. Macrolides reduce neutrophil airway inflammation with reported benefit in both eosinophilic (T2/allergic pathway) and noneosinophilic subtypes [42]. However, data in relation to asthma exacerbation and asthma phenotype that are most responsive to this mode of therapy has not been consistent across existing literature.

Gibson et al. conducted a trial investigating whether azithromycin reduces asthma exacerbations and improves quality of life in patients with symptomatic asthma treated with inhaled corticosteroid maintenance therapy [43]. This was a multicenter, randomized, double-blind, placebo-controlled, parallel group trial to evaluate the efficacy and safety of oral azithromycin 500 mg, three times weekly for 48 weeks, as add-on therapy in adults with persistent symptomatic asthma defined as asthma control score [ACQ] ≥ 0.75 despite maintenance controller therapy with an inhaled corticosteroid and a long-acting bronchodilator. Significant exclusions included: patient with >10 pack year tobacco use, parenchymal lung disease such as emphysema, DLCO <70% and prolonged QTc. Primary efficacy endpoints were the rate of total (severe and moderate) asthma exacerbations over 48 weeks and asthma quality of life. Four hundred and twenty patients were randomly assigned with equal distribution to get azithromycin or placebo. Azithromycin significantly reduced asthma exacerbations; the proportion of patients experiencing at least one asthma exacerbation was 61% patients in the placebo group versus 44% patients in the azithromycin group. In addition, azithromycin significantly improved asthma-related quality of life. Predominant side effects included diarrhea with an incidence of 34% in the azithromycin group versus 19% in the control group. The authors concluded that in adults with persistent symptomatic asthma, the addition of oral azithromycin may be a useful add-on to reduce asthma exacerbations and improve quality of life.

Bronchial Thermoplasty

Bronchial Thermoplasty (BT) is a bronchoscopic procedure in which a catheter delivers targeted radiofrequency thermal energy to the bronchial airway walls for up to 10 seconds. BT is performed as an outpatient procedure and consists of three sessions: one for the right lower lobe, one for the left lower lobe, and the last session for both upper lobes, with 3 weeks apart for each treatment. The mechanism of action involves reducing airway smooth muscle hypertrophy by partial ablation and decreasing bronchoconstriction. BT has been extensively studied in three major clinical trials, two of which have more than 5-year follow-up [44, 45].

Castro and colleagues conducted a multicenter, double-blinded, sham-controlled, randomized controlled trial (AIR2 Study) that evaluated 190 patients (18–65 years) with severe asthma randomized to BT or sham-control procedure [46]. BT improved quality of life (79% vs. 64% using AQLQ score >0.5); decreased severe exacerbations by 34%; reduced emergency room visits by 84%; and reduced time lost from work, school, and other daily activities due to asthma by 66% compared to the sham group. There was a 32% reduction rate in severe exacerbations requiring systemic steroids in the BT group compared to the sham group (0.48 vs. 0.70, 95% CI −0.031, 0.520). This effect persisted in the posttreatment period. There was no effect on lung function (FEV_1) measured by spirometry following BT. The major adverse events involved 16 patients (8.4%) in the BT group who were hospitalized for worsening of asthma symptoms, mostly on the day of the procedure. Other reported adverse effects include reversible lobar collapse, pulmonary abscess, pulmonary pseudo aneurysm, and massive hemoptysis requiring embolization.

The FDA approved BT in 2010 for severe asthma patients older than 18 years, inadequately controlled on inhaled corticosteroids and long-acting beta agonists, who can undergo bronchoscopy safely. The effectiveness of bronchial thermoplasty has been shown to persist for at least 10 years [47]. The use of BT in older adults with asthma is limited to case reports. A 70-year-old woman with refractory asthma on maximal therapy, needing frequent systemic steroids, was treated with BT and had significant systemic steroid use, lost significant weight, and had fewer exacerbations [48]. A 75-year-old man with asthma, obstructive sleep apnea, nasal polyposis, and allergic rhinitis underwent BT after multiple failed trials of medication changes. Post-BT, patient improved symptomatically and objectively, with decreased use of SABA and systemic steroid use, lost significant weight, and had fewer exacerbations [49].

In summary, BT may be offered to older adults with refractory asthma where there is expertise available.

Alternative Therapies

Herbal Medicine

Asthma has long been and continues to be treated using herbs in multiple traditional medicine systems in Europe, Middle East, India, and China, with reports of up to 80% of adults with asthma using some form of complementary medicine [50]. The exact physiological properties of herbal medicines are not fully understood, but in clinical studies, they appear to reduce airway inflammation, bronchial hyper-responsiveness, and mucus accumulation in patients with asthma. In animal models, various herbal medicines have shown evidence of reduced airway remodeling, airway inflammation, and hyper-responsiveness, likely due to COX-regulated genes exerting anti-inflammatory effects like corticosteroids [51].

While several pharmacotherapeutic agents exist for asthma symptom management leading to reduction in airway inflammation, there are several adverse effects of these agents including steroids and $\beta2$-adrenergic agonists, which may lead to patients to seek alternative therapies. In Taiwan, Chinese herbal products (CHPs) have been part of healthcare for hundreds of years and are fully reimbursed by their national health insurance. Wang et al. investigated the claims of Taiwanese health insurance database to analyze use of CHP in adults with asthma. They sampled 1 million random samples and selected ~53,000 patients with at least three outpatient asthma visits over the previous year or at least one hospitalization for asthma. Of the 24,000 adult patients with at least three outpatient asthma visits or one hospitalization for asthma over previous year, 85% were found to be users of CHP. The most commonly used CHP included Xiao-Qing-long-tang (minor green-blue dragon decoction) and ma-Xing-gan-shi-tang (ephedra, apricot kernel, licorice, and gypsum decoction) [52].

In a systematic review of the existing literature, Shergis et al. evaluated randomized controlled trials enrolling adults with asthma diagnosed based on Global Initiative of Asthma (GINA) treated with oral herbal medicine combined with add-on pharmacotherapy for at least 1 month compared with control groups including placebo only or active pharmacotherapies routinely used for asthma (corticosteroids, bronchodilators). Twenty-nine studies of low-to-moderate quality were identified, which enrolled ~3000 participants who were given herbal interventions using multiple ingredients such as licorice root, crow-dipper, astragali, and angelica. Compared with routine pharmacotherapies alone, herbal medicine as add-on therapy improved lung function (FEV1, PEFR), asthma control, reduced albuterol use, and reduced acute asthma exacerbations over 1 year. Treatment effect was higher when comparing placebo with herbal plus pharmacotherapies. The authors concluded that herbal medicines combined with routine pharmacotherapies improved asthma outcomes greater than pharmacotherapies alone but recommended additional studies given that existing ones did not blind participants, thus leading to significant possibility of bias [53].

There is limited data related to safety and efficacy of CHP in older adults. An RCT published in 2005 comparing herbal formulation ASHMI (Gang-Cao, Ku-Shen, Ling-Zhi) with prednisone 20 mg/day in adult patients aged 18–65 ($n = 94$) with moderate–persistent asthma over 4 weeks showed improved FEV_1, PEFR in both groups with statistically significant greater improvement in the prednisone group. Authors reported no significant side effects of herbal formulations [54]. Hoang et al. reported a small cohort ($n = 14$) of patients aged 22–70 with chronic refractory asthma who were treated with Sophora root for 3 years with reduced inhaled medication use and improved subjective symptom control [55].

Clinically, it is important to understand that there exists a difference in quality of these studies compared to traditional therapeutic agents as it relates to robustness of randomization, monitoring of safety parameters, and exclusion of bias. While CHP may provide some added asthma symptom control in older adults, true extent of their side effect profile is not fully understood.

Acupuncture

Acupuncture based on the "meridian theory" has been utilized to treat a variety of diseases as part of Traditional Chinese Medicine (TCM) for over 2000 years. Meridian theory was developed based upon empirical experience of relief when needling certain pulsing foci such as the medial part of lower leg for stomach aches; in total, 14 meridians were identified. The aim is to balance yin and yang energies through simulation or "needling" of these meridians or "acupoints"; newer methods include using electrical currents or lasers as opposed to needles for stimulation. According to National Institute of Health, acupuncture is increasingly employed as a complementary alternative therapy for a variety of disease states in the United States [45, 56].

Acupuncture-guided treatment of asthma is dependent on classification of asthma in TCM, typically differentiated into cold, heat, wind, stasis, and deficiency pattern/syndrome in clinic, each with a different treatment regimen incorporating acupuncture as well as other traditional Chinese therapies [57]. This methodology of diagnosis and treatment is different from allopathic medicine, and its standardization instead of customization may affect any study assessing utility of acupuncture. Pai et al. performed a cross-over study with two groups ($n = 184$, Group a and b) with mild-to-moderate asthma randomized such that one group received real acupuncture for 10 sessions followed by a washout period of 3 weeks and an additional 10 sessions of sham acupuncture, with the other group getting the same treatment in reverse order [58]. The end-points of symptom control (coughing, wheezing, dyspnea), peak flow, cell count in induced sputum (eosinophils, neutrophils), and quality of life as measured by the Questionnaire on Quality of Life Asthma (QQLA) did not show a difference between sham and real acupuncture treatment. The authors concluded that sham acupuncture cannot serve as a placebo in trials with acupuncture as the main intervention for asthma.

Additionally, caution must be exercised in interpreting asthma study results as there seem to be high levels of placebo effects in patient-reported subjective outcomes. Wechsler et al. [59] conducted a double-blind cross-over study with 46 asthmatic patients randomized to treatment with albuterol inhaler, placebo inhaler, sham acupuncture, or no intervention monitored over 12 visits. Albuterol not surprisingly increased FEV1 20% as compared with increase of 7% in other three groups; however, patient-reported outcomes did not differ significantly among albuterol inhaler (50% improvement), placebo inhaler (45%), and sham acupuncture (46%), with the no intervention control reporting only 21% improvement. Four studies have compared real acupuncture to sham acupuncture with a total of 124 participants ranging in age from 7 to 65 years [60]. The studies are limited by external validity due to a limited description of the randomization methodology, variable application of acupuncture technique, and timing of outcome assessment including immediate or up to 4 weeks later. Outcomes monitored in three of the studies were similar: lung function, bronchial responsiveness, PEFR, QOL, well-being, symptoms, and medication use. Immunological outcomes were also monitored. Only one study noted significant improvements in general well-being scores as measured by visual analog score (VAS) in the active vs. sham treatment groups; others did not notice significant differences between groups in QOL. There was improvement of immunological function as measured by IgE levels, IL-2R, and T-lymphocyte counts [60]. Significant improvements in immune function might suggest that acupuncture has a role in asthma management for some; however, again, no significant changes were identified in lung function.

Reinhold et al. evaluated the cost-effectiveness of adjunctive acupuncture compared to routine treatment alone in 306 patients investigating cost and health-related quality of life at baseline, 3 months and 6 months [61]. Acupuncture was associated with significantly higher costs primarily from the cost of sessions; however, the treatment group also had improved quality-adjusted life years. Authors concluded that acupuncture appears to be a useful and cost-effective add-on treatment. Significant side effects of acupuncture are rare, with large observational study of ~230,000 patients with 8.6% reporting any adverse effect, most commonly bleeding, nausea, and pain with 2 patients experiencing pneumothorax [62].

Review of multiple trials including meta-analysis by Martin et al. indicates that there is paucity of specific data in relation to safety and efficacy of acupuncture in older adults with asthma with mean age of 30–40 in most studies [63]. Dias et al. from 1982 included patients aged 18–73 ($n = 26$) comparing acupuncture vs control group with monitoring of PEFR which showed subjective improvement without any change in PEFR. Authors concluded that acupuncture has a placebo effect in bronchial asthma [64]. Based upon available literature, it is difficult to draw specific conclusion regarding efficacy of acupuncture in asthma treatment for older adults.

Chiropractic manipulation

Chiropractitioners view a vast array of human diseases as caused by spinal subluxations that may be corrected with spinal manipulation or adjustments including asthma [65]. The aim is to restore normal nerve function, reduce irritation of somatic and autonomic nerves by "realigning the spine" leading to mechanical (chest wall immobility) and neurological (airway tone and bronchial responsiveness) effects

[56]. Most of published data involves children and the general adult population, with no specific data in the older adult population.

Balon et al. [66] conducted a randomized partially blinded controlled trial of chiropractor spinal manipulation for children with mild-to-moderate asthma. They enrolled 91 children with persistent symptoms despite usual medical therapy randomized to active or simulated chiropractic manipulation for 4 months. The primary outcome was the change in prebronchodilator peak expiratory flow, quality of life, and symptom scores assessed at 2 and 4 months. There was a small increase in peak expiratory flow rate (7–12 L/min) from baseline in both control and treatment groups without statistical significance. Symptoms of asthma and use of beta agonists decreased, and quality of life increased in both groups. Spirometric data and airway responsiveness was unchanged. Authors concluded that in mild or moderate asthma, the addition of chiropractic spinal manipulation to usual medical care provided no benefit.

In a systematic review published in 2011, authors identified randomized trials including adult asthmatics undergoing one or more types of manual therapy, reporting clinical outcomes from EMBASE, CINAHL, MEDLINE and specialized database for complementary medicine including Index of Chiropractic Literature (ICL) and MANTIS. Three RCTs were identified from 68 full text articles; data could not be pooled due to disparate patient groups and outcomes. Only two of these trials investigated chiropractic spinal manipulation with a sham maneuver, and neither trial found significant difference. Authors concluded there is insufficient evidence to support the use of manual therapies for patients with asthma, and there is a need for adequately sized RCTs that examine the effects of manual therapy on clinically relevant outcomes [67]. Eight articles met the inclusion criteria of this review in the form of one case series, one case study, one survey, two randomized controlled trials (RCTs), one randomized patient and observer blinded cross-over trial, one single blind cross-study design, and one self-reported impairment questionnaire. Based upon inclusion of weak levels of evidence, authors concluded that chiropractic care showed improvements in subjective measures of asthma and, to a lesser degree objective measures, none of which were statistically significant [68].

Chiropractors have largely pointed to anecdotal evidence in support of asthma benefit, but no large randomized trials or meta-analysis of published literature has supported this conclusion. The level of evidence supporting use of chiropractic manipulation as treatment of asthma is weak or insufficient, and there is a need for adequately sized RCTs to examine the effects of manual therapy on clinically relevant and objective outcomes. In regard to the older adult population, special care should be used, especially in older patient's dependent on oral corticosteroids or with other risk factors for osteoporosis due to the high risk of fractures associated with spinal manipulation.

Yoga

Yoga is considered by practitioners to be the union of body and mind. There are different types of yoga from physical movements to mindful mediation. Pranayama is a form of yoga with a series of breathing exercises. The effects of pranayama were evaluated in 50 asthma patients with mild-to-moderate severity. Subjects were allocated to a treatment group (who practices 5 series of breathing exercises for 20 minutes twice daily for 12 weeks) and a control group who were practicing meditation for 20 minutes twice daily for 12 weeks. Lung function tests such as FEV_1 and peak expiratory flow (PEFR) were assessed pre-and post- 12 weeks. After 12 weeks, the treatment group had improved FEV_1 and PEFR compared to the control group.

Vempati and colleagues conducted an open-label randomized placebo control trial of yoga in patients with mild-to-moderate asthma [69]. The experimental group underwent comprehensive yoga-based lifestyle modifications and a stress management program for 4 hours a day for 2 weeks with an additional 4 weeks practice at home. The control group received conventional care. Fifty-seven subjects completed the study (Yoga group, $n = 29$ and control group, $n = 28$). They found statistically significant improvements in FEV_1, PEFR, and reduced exercise-induced bronchoconstriction in the yoga group compared to control. Both groups had improved AQOL; however, the yoga group achieved the above improvements earlier and it was sustained. The frequency of rescue medication use was lower in both groups. There was no significant change in serum eosinophil cationic protein. The authors were unsure of the mechanism of action for improvements in asthma outcomes with yoga.

Yang and colleagues published a Cochrane review of 15 randomized control trials with 1048 participants with mild-to-moderate asthma [70]. Five studies include yoga breathing alone, while other studies included yoga breathing, posture, and meditation. Interventions lasted from 2 weeks to 54 months, and for no more than 6 months in most studies. There was statistically significant evidence that yoga improves quality of life (AQLQ score), symptoms, and reduces medication use in people with asthma. There was a statistically significant change in lung function measured by FEV_1. No serious adverse events were reported. There was moderate-quality evidence that yoga may lead to small improvements in quality of life and symptoms in people with asthma. There is need for large randomized studies to confirm the effects of yoga for asthma. There is paucity of data on yoga in older adults with asthma.

Conclusions

Data on safety and efficacy of novel and alternative therapies in asthma are available in the younger adult population, and only scarce data or studies target the older asthma population. Furthermore, the long-term safety profile of such therapies in older asthmatic patients is nonexistent. Omalizumab and mepolizumab have been evaluated in small studies in older patients with severe asthma, and appear to be well tolerated and effective. Data from other existing biologics are not available for older patients with asthma. Alternatives methods have been evaluated in asthma with limited evidence and mixed benefit results.

References

1. World's older population grows dramatically, March 28, 2016. https://www.nih.gov/news-events/news-releases/worlds-older-population-grows-dramatically.
2. Wan He DG, Kowal P. An Aging world: 2015, international population report, Census.gov, P95/16-1, March 2016.
3. Akinbami LJ, Moorman JE, Liu X. Asthma prevalence, health care use, and mortality: United States, 2005–2009. Natl Health Stat Rep. 2011;(32):1–14.
4. Yanez A, Cho SH, Soriano JB, Rosenwasser LJ, Rodrigo GJ, Rabe KF, et al. Asthma in the elderly: what we know and what we have yet to know. World Allergy Organ J. 2014;7(1):8.
5. Skloot GS, Busse PJ, Braman SS, Kovacs EJ, Dixon AE, Vaz Fragoso CA, et al. An Official American Thoracic Society workshop report: evaluation and management of asthma in the elderly. Ann Am Thorac Soc. 2016;13(11):2064–77.
6. Chung KF. Managing severe asthma in adults: lessons from the ERS/ATS guidelines. Curr Opin Pulm Med. 2015;21(1):8–15.
7. Lindsay JT, Heaney LG. Non-adherence in difficult asthma and advances in detection. Expert Rev Respir Med. 2013;7(6):607–14.
8. Corren J, Casale T, Deniz Y, Ashby M. Omalizumab, a recombinant humanized anti-IgE antibody, reduces asthma-related emergency room visits and hospitalizations in patients with allergic asthma. J Allergy Clin Immunol. 2003;111(1):87–90.
9. Hanania NA, Wenzel S, Rosen K, Hsieh HJ, Mosesova S, Choy DF, et al. Exploring the effects of omalizumab in allergic asthma: an analysis of biomarkers in the EXTRA study. Am J Respir Crit Care Med. 2013;187(8):804–11.
10. Hammond C, Kurten M, Kennedy JL. Rhinovirus and asthma: a storied history of incompatibility. Curr Allergy Asthma Rep. 2015;15(2):502.
11. Esquivel A, Busse WW, Calatroni A, Togias AG, Grindle KG, Bochkov YA, et al. Effects of omalizumab on rhinovirus infections, illnesses, and exacerbations of asthma. Am J Respir Crit Care Med. 2017;196(8):985–92.
12. Humbert M, Busse W, Hanania NA, Lowe PJ, Canvin J, Erpenbeck VJ, et al. Omalizumab in asthma: an update on recent developments. J Allergy Clin Immunol Pract. 2014;2(5):525–36.e1.
13. Kim HL, Leigh R, Omalizumab BA. Practical considerations regarding the risk of anaphylaxis. Allergy Asthma Clin Immunol. 2010;6(1):32.
14. Sposato B, Scalese M, Latorre M, Scichilone N, Matucci A, Milanese M, et al. Effects of omalizumab in severe asthmatics across ages: A real life Italian experience. Respir Med. 2016;119:141–9.
15. Maykut RJ, Kianifard F, Geba GP. Response of older patients with IgE-mediated asthma to omalizumab: a pooled analysis. J Asthma. 2008;45(3):173–81.
16. Tat TS, Cilli A. Evaluation of long-term safety and efficacy of omalizumab in elderly patients with uncontrolled allergic asthma. Ann Allergy Asthma Immunol. 2016;117(5):546–9.
17. Wallen N, Kita H, Weiler D, Gleich GJ. Glucocorticoids inhibit cytokine-mediated eosinophil survival. J Immunol (Baltimore, Md: 1950). 1991;147(10):3490–5.
18. Pavord ID, Korn S, Howarth P, Bleecker ER, Buhl R, Keene ON, et al. Mepolizumab for severe eosinophilic asthma (DREAM): a multicentre, double-blind, placebo-controlled trial. Lancet (London, England). 2012;380(9842):651–9.
19. Ortega HG, Liu MC, Pavord ID, Brusselle GG, FitzGerald JM, Chetta A, et al. Mepolizumab treatment in patients with severe eosinophilic asthma. N Engl J Med. 2014;371(13):1198–207.
20. Hector Ortega BM, Yancey S. Rohit Katial, Response to treatment with mepolizumab in elderly patients. Americal Journal of Respiratory and Critical care Medicine 2015;191:A4177.
21. Bel EH, Wenzel SE, Thompson PJ, Prazma CM, Keene ON, Yancey SW, et al. Oral glucocorticoid-sparing effect of mepolizumab in eosinophilic asthma. N Engl J Med. 2014;371(13):1189–97.

22. Khatri S, Moore W, Gibson PG, Leigh R, Bourdin A, Maspero J, et al. Assessment of the long-term safety of mepolizumab and durability of clinical response in patients with severe eosinophilic asthma. J Allergy Clin Immunol. 2019;143(5):1742–51.
23. Lugogo N, Domingo C, Chanez P, Leigh R, Gilson MJ, Price RG, et al. Long-term efficacy and safety of mepolizumab in patients with severe eosinophilic asthma: a multi-center, open-label, phase IIIb study. Clin Ther. 2016;38(9):2058–70.e1.
24. Egan RW, Athwal D, Bodmer MW, Carter JM, Chapman RW, Chou CC, et al. Effect of Sch 55700, a humanized monoclonal antibody to human interleukin-5, on eosinophilic responses and bronchial hyperreactivity. Arzneimittelforschung. 1999;49(9):779–90.
25. Kips JC, O'Connor BJ, Langley SJ, Woodcock A, Kerstjens HA, Postma DS, et al. Effect of SCH55700, a humanized anti-human interleukin-5 antibody, in severe persistent asthma: a pilot study. Am J Respir Crit Care Med. 2003;167(12):1655–9.
26. Castro M, Mathur S, Hargreave F, Boulet LP, Xie F, Young J, et al. Reslizumab for poorly controlled, eosinophilic asthma: a randomized, placebo-controlled study. Am J Respir Crit Care Med. 2011;184(10):1125–32.
27. Castro M, Zangrilli J, Wechsler ME. Corrections. Reslizumab for inadequately controlled asthma with elevated blood eosinophil counts: results from two multicentre, parallel, double-blind, randomised, placebo-controlled, phase 3 trials. Lancet Respir Med. 2015;3(4):e15.
28. Brusselle G, Germinaro M, Weiss S, Zangrilli J. Reslizumab in patients with inadequately controlled late-onset asthma and elevated blood eosinophils. Pulm Pharmacol Ther. 2017;43:39–45.
29. Bjermer L, Lemiere C, Maspero J, Weiss S, Zangrilli J, Germinaro M. Reslizumab for inadequately controlled asthma with elevated blood eosinophil levels: a randomized phase 3 study. Chest. 2016;150(4):789–98.
30. Sahota J, Robinson DS. Update on new biologics for intractable eosinophilic asthma: impact of reslizumab. Drug Des Devel Ther. 2018;12:1173–81.
31. Gour N, Wills-Karp M. IL-4 and IL-13 signaling in allergic airway disease. Cytokine. 2015;75(1):68–78.
32. Laviolette M, Gossage DL, Gauvreau G, Leigh R, Olivenstein R, Katial R, et al. Effects of benralizumab on airway eosinophils in asthmatic patients with sputum eosinophilia. J Allergy Clin Immunol. 2013;132(5):1086–96.e5.
33. Sastre J, Davila I. Dupilumab: a new paradigm for the treatment of allergic diseases. J Investig Allergol Clin Immunol. 2018;28(3):139–50.
34. Nowak RM, Parker JM, Silverman RA, Rowe BH, Smithline H, Khan F, et al. A randomized trial of benralizumab, an antiinterleukin 5 receptor alpha monoclonal antibody, after acute asthma. Am J Emerg Med. 2015;33(1):14–20.
35. Castro M, Wenzel SE, Bleecker ER, Pizzichini E, Kuna P, Busse WW, et al. Benralizumab, an anti-interleukin 5 receptor alpha monoclonal antibody, versus placebo for uncontrolled eosinophilic asthma: a phase 2b randomised dose-ranging study. Lancet Respir Med. 2014;2(11):879–90.
36. FitzGerald JM, Bleecker ER, Nair P, Korn S, Ohta K, Lommatzsch M, et al. Benralizumab, an anti-interleukin-5 receptor alpha monoclonal antibody, as add-on treatment for patients with severe, uncontrolled, eosinophilic asthma (CALIMA): a randomised, double-blind, placebo-controlled phase 3 trial. Lancet (London, England). 2016;388(10056):2128–41.
37. Bleecker ER, FitzGerald JM, Chanez P, Papi A, Weinstein SF, Barker P, et al. Efficacy and safety of benralizumab for patients with severe asthma uncontrolled with high-dosage inhaled corticosteroids and long-acting beta2-agonists (SIROCCO): a randomised, multicentre, placebo-controlled phase 3 trial. Lancet (London, England). 2016;388(10056):2115–27.
38. Nair P, Wenzel S, Rabe KF, Bourdin A, Lugogo NL, Kuna P, et al. Oral glucocorticoid-sparing effect of benralizumab in severe asthma. N Engl J Med. 2017;376(25):2448–58.
39. Wenzel S, Ford L, Pearlman D, Spector S, Sher L, Skobieranda F, et al. Dupilumab in persistent asthma with elevated eosinophil levels. N Engl J Med. 2013;368(26):2455–66.
40. Castro M, Corren J, Pavord ID, Maspero J, Wenzel S, Rabe KF, et al. Dupilumab efficacy and safety in moderate-to-severe uncontrolled asthma. N Engl J Med. 2018;378(26):2486–96.

41. Rabe KF, Nair P, Brusselle G, Maspero JF, Castro M, Sher L, et al. Efficacy and safety of dupilumab in glucocorticoid-dependent severe asthma. N Engl J Med. 2018;378(26):2475–85.
42. Brusselle GG, Vanderstichele C, Jordens P, Deman R, Slabbynck H, Ringoet V, et al. Azithromycin for prevention of exacerbations in severe asthma (AZISAST): a multicentre randomised double-blind placebo-controlled trial. Thorax. 2013;68(4):322–9.
43. Gibson PG, Yang IA, Upham JW, Reynolds PN, Hodge S, James AL, et al. Effect of azithromycin on asthma exacerbations and quality of life in adults with persistent uncontrolled asthma (AMAZES): a randomised, double-blind, placebo-controlled trial. Lancet (London, England). 2017;390(10095):659–68.
44. Castro M, Rubin A, Laviolette M, Hanania NA, Armstrong B, Cox G. Persistence of effectiveness of bronchial thermoplasty in patients with severe asthma. Ann Allergy Asthma Immunology. 2011;107(1):65–70.
45. Zhou W, Benharash P. Effects and mechanisms of acupuncture based on the principle of meridians. J Acupunct Meridian Stud. 2014;7(4):190–3.
46. Castro M, Rubin AS, Laviolette M, Fiterman J, De Andrade Lima M, Shah PL, et al. Effectiveness and safety of bronchial thermoplasty in the treatment of severe asthma: a multicenter, randomized, double-blind, sham-controlled clinical trial. Am J Respir Crit Care Med. 2010;181(2):116–24.
47. Tan LD, Yoneda KY, Louie S, Hogarth DK, Castro M. Bronchial thermoplasty: a decade of experience: state of the art. J Allergy Clin Immunol Pract. 2019;7(1):71–80.
48. Minami D, Ando C, Nakasuka T, Iwamoto Y, Sato K, Fujiwara K, et al. Usefulness of bronchial thermoplasty for patients with a deteriorating lung function. Intern Med (Tokyo, Japan). 2018;57(1):75–9.
49. Tolla AS, El-Zein RS, Saludes M. Bronchial thermoplasty in an elderly severely asthmatic patient with obstructive sleep apnea. J Bronchol Interv Pulmonol. 2018;25(4):e51–e2.
50. Ziment I, Tashkin DP. Alternative medicine for allergy and asthma. J Allergy Clin Immunol. 2000;106(4):603–14.
51. Lim YJ, Na HS, Yun YS, Choi IS, Oh JS, Rhee JH, et al. Suppressive effects of ginsan on the development of allergic reaction in murine asthmatic model. Int Arch Allergy Immunol. 2009;150(1):32–42.
52. Wang HM, Lin SK, Yeh CH, Lai JN. Prescription pattern of Chinese herbal products for adult-onset asthma in Taiwan: a population-based study. Ann Allergy Asthma Immunol. 2014;112(5):465–70.
53. Shergis JL, Wu L, Zhang AL, Guo X, Lu C, Xue CC. Herbal medicine for adults with asthma: a systematic review. J Asthma. 2016;53(6):650–9.
54. Wen MC, Wei CH, Hu ZQ, Srivastava K, Ko J, Xi ST, et al. Efficacy and tolerability of antiasthma herbal medicine intervention in adult patients with moderate-severe allergic asthma. J Allergy Clin Immunol. 2005;116(3):517–24.
55. Hoang BX, Shaw DG, Levine S, Hoang C, Pham P. New approach in asthma treatment using excitatory modulator. Phytother Res. 2007;21(6):554–7.
56. Markham AW, Wilkinson JM. Complementary and alternative medicines (CAM) in the management of asthma: an examination of the evidence. J Asthma. 2004;41(2):131–9.
57. Zheng LB. Professor LIN Lin's clinical experiences of comprehensive internal and external therapy for asthma. Zhongguo Zhen Jiu. 2013;33(5):447–50.
58. Pai HJ, Azevedo RS, Braga AL, Martins LC, Saraiva-Romanholo BM, Martins Mde A, et al. A randomized, controlled, crossover study in patients with mild and moderate asthma undergoing treatment with traditional Chinese acupuncture. Clinics (Sao Paulo, Brazil). 2015;70(10):663–9.
59. Wechsler ME, Kelley JM, Boyd IO, Dutile S, Marigowda G, Kirsch I, et al. Active albuterol or placebo, sham acupuncture, or no intervention in asthma. N Engl J Med. 2011;365(2):119–26.
60. Yang YQ, Chen HP, Wang Y, Yin LM, Xu YD, Ran J. Considerations for use of acupuncture as supplemental therapy for patients with allergic asthma. Clin Rev Allergy Immunol. 2013;44(3):254–61.

61. Reinhold T, Brinkhaus B, Willich SN, Witt C. Acupuncture in patients suffering from allergic asthma: is it worth additional costs? J Altern Complement Med (New York, NY). 2014;20(3):169–77.
62. MacPherson H, Thomas K, Walters S, Fitter M. A prospective survey of adverse events and treatment reactions following 34,000 consultations with professional acupuncturists. Acupunct Medicine. 2001;19(2):93–102.
63. Martin J, Donaldson AN, Villarroel R, Parmar MK, Ernst E, Higginson IJ. Efficacy of acupuncture in asthma: systematic review and meta-analysis of published data from 11 randomised controlled trials. Eur Respir J. 2002;20(4):846–52.
64. Dias PL, Subramaniam S, Lionel ND. Effects of acupuncture in bronchial asthma: preliminary communication. J R Soc Med. 1982;75(4):245–8.
65. Ernst E. Chiropractic treatment for asthma? J Asthma. 2009;46(3):211.
66. Balon J, Aker PD, Crowther ER, Danielson C, Cox PG, O'Shaughnessy D, et al. A comparison of active and simulated chiropractic manipulation as adjunctive treatment for childhood asthma. N Engl J Med. 1998;339(15):1013–20.
67. Hondras MA, Linde K, Jones AP. Manual therapy for asthma. Cochrane Database Syst Rev. 2005;(2):CD001002.
68. Kaminskyj A, Frazier M, Johnstone K, Gleberzon BJ. Chiropractic care for patients with asthma: a systematic review of the literature. J Can Chiropr Assoc. 2010;54(1):24–32.
69. Vempati R, Bijlani RL, Deepak KK. The efficacy of a comprehensive lifestyle modification programme based on yoga in the management of bronchial asthma: a randomized controlled trial. BMC Pulm Med. 2009;9:37.
70. Yang ZY, Zhong HB, Mao C, Yuan JQ, Huang YF, Wu XY, et al. Yoga for asthma. Cochrane Database Syst Rev. 2016;4:Cd010346.

Index

© Springer Nature Switzerland AG 2019
T. E. G. Epstein, S. M. Nyenhuis (eds.), *Treatment of Asthma in Older Adults*,
https://doi.org/10.1007/978-3-030-20554-6

Printed in the United States
By Bookmasters